FOCUSING ON CHILDREN'S HEALTH
Community Approaches to Addressing Health Disparities

Workshop Summary

Theresa M. Wizemann and Karen M. Anderson, *Rapporteurs*

Roundtable on Health Disparities

Board on Population Health and Public Health Practice

Board on Children, Youth, and Families

INSTITUTE OF MEDICINE *AND*
NATIONAL RESEARCH COUNCIL
OF THE NATIONAL ACADEMIES

THE NATIONAL ACADEMIES PRESS
Washington, D.C.
www.nap.edu

THE NATIONAL ACADEMIES PRESS   500 Fifth Street, N.W.   Washington, DC 20001

NOTICE: The project that is the subject of this report was approved by the Governing Board of the National Research Council, whose members are drawn from the councils of the National Academy of Sciences, the National Academy of Engineering, and the Institute of Medicine.

This study was supported by multiple contracts and grants between the National Academy of Sciences and the Agency for Healthcare Research and Quality (Contract HHSP23320042509XI, TO#11), California Endowment (Contract 20052634), California Health Care Foundation (Contract 06-1213), Commonwealth Fund (Contract 20060048), Connecticut Health Foundation (unnumbered grant), Ford Foundation (Contract 1050-0152,FF5H003), Healthcare Georgia Foundation (unnumbered grant), the Henry J. Kaiser Family Foundation (Contract 01-1149-810), Kaiser Permanente (Contract 20072164), Merck (unnumbered grant), Missouri Foundation for Health (Contract 06-0022-HPC), Robert Wood Johnson Foundation (Contract 56387), and the W.K. Kellogg Foundation (Contract P0123822). Any opinions, findings, conclusions, or recommendations expressed in this publication are those of the author(s) and do not necessarily reflect the view of the organizations or agencies that provided support for this project.

International Standard Book Number-13:   978-0-309-13785-0
International Standard Book Number-10:   0-309-13785-3

Additional copies of this report are available from the National Academies Press, 500 Fifth Street, N.W., Lockbox 285, Washington, DC 20055; (800) 624-6242 or (202) 334-3313 (in the Washington metropolitan area); Internet, http://www.nap. edu.

For more information about the Institute of Medicine, visit the IOM home page at: **www.iom.edu.**

Printed in the United States of America

The serpent has been a symbol of long life, healing, and knowledge among almost all cultures and religions since the beginning of recorded history. The serpent adopted as a logotype by the Institute of Medicine is a relief carving from ancient Greece, now held by the Staatliche Museen in Berlin.

Suggested citation: IOM (Institute of Medicine). 2009. *Focusing on children's health: Community approaches to addressing health disparities: Workshop summary.* Washington, DC: The National Academies Press.

"Knowing is not enough; we must apply.
Willing is not enough; we must do."

—Goethe

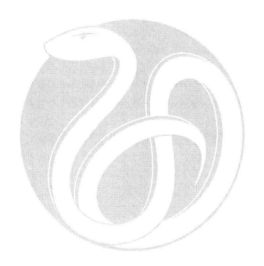

INSTITUTE OF MEDICINE
OF THE NATIONAL ACADEMIES

Advising the Nation. Improving Health.

THE NATIONAL ACADEMIES
Advisers to the Nation on Science, Engineering, and Medicine

The **National Academy of Sciences** is a private, nonprofit, self-perpetuating society of distinguished scholars engaged in scientific and engineering research, dedicated to the furtherance of science and technology and to their use for the general welfare. Upon the authority of the charter granted to it by the Congress in 1863, the Academy has a mandate that requires it to advise the federal government on scientific and technical matters. Dr. Ralph J. Cicerone is president of the National Academy of Sciences.

The **National Academy of Engineering** was established in 1964, under the charter of the National Academy of Sciences, as a parallel organization of outstanding engineers. It is autonomous in its administration and in the selection of its members, sharing with the National Academy of Sciences the responsibility for advising the federal government. The National Academy of Engineering also sponsors engineering programs aimed at meeting national needs, encourages education and research, and recognizes the superior achievements of engineers. Dr. Charles M. Vest is president of the National Academy of Engineering.

The **Institute of Medicine** was established in 1970 by the National Academy of Sciences to secure the services of eminent members of appropriate professions in the examination of policy matters pertaining to the health of the public. The Institute acts under the responsibility given to the National Academy of Sciences by its congressional charter to be an adviser to the federal government and, upon its own initiative, to identify issues of medical care, research, and education. Dr. Harvey V. Fineberg is president of the Institute of Medicine.

The **National Research Council** was organized by the National Academy of Sciences in 1916 to associate the broad community of science and technology with the Academy's purposes of furthering knowledge and advising the federal government. Functioning in accordance with general policies determined by the Academy, the Council has become the principal operating agency of both the National Academy of Sciences and the National Academy of Engineering in providing services to the government, the public, and the scientific and engineering communities. The Council is administered jointly by both Academies and the Institute of Medicine. Dr. Ralph J. Cicerone and Dr. Charles M. Vest are chair and vice chair, respectively, of the National Research Council.

www.national-academies.org

ROUNDTABLE ON HEALTH DISPARITIES[1]

Nicole Lurie (*Chair*), Senior Natural Scientist, RAND Corporation, Arlington, VA

Victoria H. Barbosa, President, Dermal Insights, Inc., Chicago, IL

Anne C. Beal, Senior Program Officer, Quality of Care of Underserved Population, Commonwealth Fund, New York

Cheryl A. Boyce, Executive Director, Ohio Commission on Minority Health, Vern Riffe Center for Government and the Performing Arts, Columbus, OH

America Bracho, CEO, Latino Health Access, Anaheim, CA

Francis D. Chesley, Director, Office of Extramural Research, Education, and Priority Populations, Agency for Healthcare Research and Quality, Rockville, MD

Todd Cox, Program Officer, Racial Justice and Minority Rights, Ford Foundation, New York

William F. Crimi, Vice President, Program and Evaluation, Connecticut Health Foundation, New Britain, CT

Alicia Dixon, Program Officer, The California Endowment, Los Angeles

José J. Escarce, Professor of Medicine, David Geffen School of Medicine, University of California, Los Angeles

Garth N. Graham, Deputy Assistant Secretary, Minority Health Department of Health and Human Services, Office of Minority Health, Rockville, MD

Tom Granatir, Director, Policy and Communications, Innovation Center Humana, Inc., Chicago, IL

Cara V. James, Senior Policy Analyst, Henry J. Kaiser Family Foundation, Washington, DC

Jennie R. Joe, Professor, Department of Family and Community Medicine, and Director, NARTC, University of Arizona, College of Medicine, Tucson, AZ

James R. Kimmey, President and CEO, Missouri Foundation for Health, St. Louis

Howard K. Koh, Associate Dean and Director, Division of Public Health Practice, Harvard School of Public Health, Boston, MA

James Krieger, Chief, Epidemiology Planning and Evaluation Unit, Seattle, WA

Anne C. Kubisch, Codirector, Roundtable on Community Change, Aspen Institute, New York

---

[1] IOM forums and roundtables do not issue, review, or approve individual documents. The responsibility for the published workshop summary rests with the workshop rapporteurs and the institution.

Study Staff

Karen M. Anderson, Senior Program Officer *(April 2008 through present)*
Jennifer A. Cohen, Program Officer *(July 2007 through April 2008)*
Rose Marie Martinez, Board Director
Thelma L. Cox, Senior Program Assistant *(April 2008 through January 2009)*
Pamela Lighter, Program Assistant *(February 2009 through present)*
Patrick Burke, Financial Officer
Hope Hare, Administrative Assistant
Yi Cai, Intern *(May 2009 through July 2009)*

Reviewers

This report has been reviewed in draft form by individuals chosen for their diverse perspectives and technical expertise, in accordance with procedures approved by the National Research Council's Report Review Committee. The purpose of this independent review is to provide candid and critical comments that will assist the institution in making its published report as sound as possible and to ensure that the report meets institutional standards for objectivity, evidence, and responsiveness to the study charge. The review comments and draft manuscript remain confidential to protect the integrity of the deliberative process. We wish to thank the following individuals for their review of this report:

Maxine Hayes, Department of Health, Washington
Cara James, Kaiser Family Foundation
Barbara Starfield, Johns Hopkins University

Although the reviewers listed above have provided many constructive comments and suggestions, they were not asked to endorse the final draft of the report before its release. The review of this report was overseen by **Dr. Bobbie Berkowitz.** Appointed by the Institute of Medicine, she was responsible for making certain that an independent examination of this report was carried out in accordance with institutional procedures and that all review comments were carefully considered. Responsibility for the final content of this report rests entirely with the rapporteurs and the institution.

Contents

Tables, Figures, and Boxes

TABLES

FIGURES

BOXES

Preface

In early 2007, the Institute of Medicine (IOM) of the National Academies convened the Roundtable on Health Disparities to increase the visibility of racial and ethnic health disparities as a national problem, further the development of programs and strategies to reduce disparities, and track promising activities and developments in health care that could lead to dramatically reducing or eliminating disparities. The Roundtable on Health Disparities includes representatives from the health professions, state and local government, foundations, philanthropy, academia, advocacy groups, and community-based organizations. Its mission is to facilitate communication across sectors and—above all—to generate action. Through national and local activities, the Roundtable strives to advance the goal of eliminating health disparities.

On January 24, 2008, the Roundtable on Health Disparities, in collaboration with the Board on Children, Youth, and Families of the National Research Council and the IOM, held a workshop at the Morehouse School of Medicine's Louis W. Sullivan National Center for Primary Care Auditorium in Atlanta, Georgia. The Roundtable brought together a diverse group of experts from a variety of fields to discuss the relationship between socioeconomic conditions early in life and later health outcomes. Life course epidemiology has added a further dimension to our understanding of the social determinants of health by showing an association between early socioeconomic conditions and adult health related behaviors as well as adult morbidity and mortality. Realizing that the foundations of adult health and adult health behaviors are laid prenatally and early in childhood, the Roundtable's workshop focused on (1) describing the evidence linking early childhood life conditions and adult health outcomes; (2) discussing the contribution of early childhood conditions to observed racial and ethnic disparities in health; (3) highlighting successful models that engage both community factors and health care factors that affect life course development; and (4) facilitating discussion of these issues among stakeholders in academia, community development, health care, business, and philanthropy.

The workshop provided the Roundtable members with an opportunity to hear from a diverse set of people from across the country and to engage in an open dialogue about the relevant issues and concerns related to reducing health disparities. Additionally, workshop attendees offered differing perspectives and unique approaches to these issues. Together, research, experiences, evidence, and knowledge were shared across the two groups.

ACKNOWLEDGMENTS

The Roundtable on Health Disparities thanks all workshop participants for their individual contributions to this workshop. Their willingness to share their time and expertise led to frank discussions about the long-term effects of social conditions during childhood.

We especially want to extend thanks to Dr. David Satcher of the Morehouse School of Medicine and his staff for sponsoring and hosting the workshop in the Louis W. Sullivan National Center for Primary Care Auditorium. Deborah Jones, in particular, was incredibly helpful at every step of the way as we organized the workshop.

We are also indebted to Dr. Gary Nelson and Janette Blackburn from the Healthcare Georgia Foundation for sponsoring this workshop and for assisting with all aspects of the workshop planning.

We also want to thank Dr. Charles Bruner and Dr. Edward Schor for their collaboration on the background paper that was commissioned by the Roundtable for this workshop. Their paper, "Clinical Health Care Practice and Community Building: Addressing Racial Disparities in Healthy Child Development," is in Appendix E. We also want to thank Dr. Bernard Guyer for sharing his paper "Investments to Promote Children's Health: A Systematic Literature Review and Economic Analysis of Interventions in the Preschool Period" with the Roundtable. Biosketches for all presenters are in Appendix B.

The Roundtable also thanks IOM staff for their ongoing efforts to support the work of the Roundtable. Sincere gratitude is extended to Dr. Rose Marie Martinez, Director of the Board on Population Health and Public Health Practice; Jennifer Cohen, for planning, organizing, and implementing this workshop; and Thelma Cox for managing all of the administrative components of the meeting. We also want to extend thanks to Christie Bell and Hope Hare for their ongoing assistance and support.

Finally, special thanks to all of the sponsors who make the Roundtable on Health Disparities a reality. Financial support for the Roundtable and its activities was provided by the Agency for Healthcare Research and Quality in HHS; the Office of Minority Health in HHS; the California Endowment, the California Health Care Foundation; the Commonwealth Fund; the Connecticut Health Foundation; the Ford Foundation; the Healthcare Georgia Foundation; the Henry J. Kaiser Family Foundation; Kaiser Permanente; Merck; the Missouri Foundation for Health; the Robert Wood Johnson Foundation; and the W.K. Kellogg Foundation.

Dr. Nicole Lurie, *Chair*
Roundtable on Health Disparities

1

Introduction

Socioeconomic conditions are known to be major determinants of health at all stages of life, from pregnancy through childhood and adulthood. "Life-course epidemiology" has added a further dimension to the understanding of the social determinants of health by showing an association between early-life socioeconomic conditions and adult health-related behaviors, morbidity, and mortality. Sensitive and critical periods of development, such as the prenatal period and early childhood, present significant opportunities to influence lifelong health. Yet simply intervening in the health system is insufficient to influence health early in the life course. Community-level approaches to affect key determinants of health are also critical. Many of these issues were raised in the 1995 National Academies report *Children's Health, the Nation's Wealth: Assessing and Improving Child Health*. The present workshop builds upon this earlier report with presentations and examples from the field.

In his welcome address to the workshop participants, John E. Maupin, Jr., of the Morehouse School of Medicine expressed optimism that both the health care delivery system and the health status of children can be improved, and perhaps more importantly, a culture of wellness can be created in communities by educating parents and fostering prevention.

Gary Nelson, of the Healthcare Georgia Foundation, noted that the workshop program was grounded in science, built on partnerships, and focused on results. Nelson said that the workshop holds a special significance for the host city, Atlanta, for the state of Georgia, and for the southeast region, as they know firsthand the effect of the enduring gaps in education, health, income, and opportunity.

SCOPE OF THE WORKSHOP

On January 24, 2008, the Institute of Medicine's Roundtable on Health Disparities; the Institute of Medicine's Board on Children, Youth, and Families; the Satcher Health Leadership Institute of the Morehouse School of Medicine; and the Healthcare Georgia Foundation cosponsored a public workshop to discuss in depth the important foundations of adult health that are laid prenatally and early in childhood. Nicole Lurie, chair of the IOM Roundtable, noted that those who study the health care system and those who study social determinants of health do not have many opportunities to interact with one another, either on an academic level or on a community level. As such, the workshop, entitled "Investing in Children's Health: A Community Approach to Addressing Health Disparities," was designed to continue to advance the dialogue about health disparities by facilitating discussion among stakeholders in the community, academia, health care, business, policy, and philanthropy.

Workshop speakers were asked to do the following:

- Describe the evidence linking early childhood life conditions and adult health.
- Discuss the contribution of the early life course to observed racial and ethnic disparities in health.
- Highlight successful models that engage both community factors and health care to affect life course development.

David Satcher, 16th surgeon general of the United States and director of the Satcher Health Leadership Institute, presented the keynote address to the Roundtable, describing investments in children's health and how policy can affect children's lives. The foundation for discussion was then set by the presentation of two review papers, one by Bernard Guyer of the Johns Hopkins Bloomberg School of Public Health, analyzing the economics of early childhood interventions, and one by Charles Bruner of the Child Family Policy Center and Edward Schor of the Commonwealth Fund, addressing clinical practice and community building. The practical issues of implementing health policies directed toward children were discussed by Christine Ferguson of the George Washington University Department of Heath Policy and Yvonne Sanders-Butler of Browns Mill Elementary and Magnet School in Georgia.

Mildred Thompson of PolicyLink and co-chair of the Roundtable provided the workshop participants with an opportunity to preview a segment of a forthcoming PBS documentary series entitled *Unnatural Causes: Is Inequality Making Us Sick?*, which explores socioeconomic and racial inequities in health. The segment screened at the workshop, entitled "When the

Bough Breaks," addressed the disproportionate infant mortality rates and preterm births of African American women. The video and the discussion that followed are discussed in greater detail in Appendix D.

Examples of community development approaches in the host city, Atlanta, were discussed by Veda Johnson of Emory University School of Medicine; Marshall Kreuter, Roddie Longino, and Travie Leslie of Georgia State University; and Wayne Giles of the Centers for Disease Control and Prevention (CDC). Finally, the role of the business sector in improving communities and fostering health was discussed by Sandra White of WellPoint, Inc., Michelle Courton Brown of Bank of America, and Maureen Kelly of the ING Foundation.

KEY THEMES

Throughout the day, workshop participants highlighted several recurring themes:

- Action: The roles of social, racial, and economic determinants of health are well known. Several participants noted that although continued documentation and analysis of disparities is still needed, what is really needed now is action. The success of model programs shows that disparities in health are not insurmountable.

- Circular: Workshop participants discussed the social, environmental, economic, and genetic influences that affect the health of a child. The health status of the child, in turn, affects total child development and well-being, including education, social development, economic welfare, and justice.

- Community involvement: Speakers and workshop participants alike noted that successful interventions involve the community as a full partner in the process. Identification of health challenges and priority concerns, and the development of intervention strategies suited to a community's needs and culture, cannot be done without the input of the community members.

- Coordination: As described by several presenters, there are many effective strategies in use in communities throughout the country. However, they further stated that there is a need for a more nationally coordinated effort, moving beyond individuals and communities, to systems-level change. Information about successful models needs to be disseminated so resources are not wasted through creating same or similar interventions anew from program to program.

- Communication: Workshop participants discussed the need for better communication in order to foster communication among all people and organizations involved in addressing health disparities, including among and within government agencies. A clear, carefully framed message, with supporting data where possible, is needed to convey the importance of addressing disparities to policy makers and to gain their support of programs.

- Sustainability: Finally, speakers and workshop attendees repeatedly raised the issue of grant funding, philanthropy, and government programs that provide a limited amount of funding for a finite period of time, often only a few years. A role for sustainable funding sources was described in the workshop as being critical in achieving nationwide, multigenerational success in eliminating health disparities.

ORGANIZATION OF THE REPORT

The report that follows summarizes the presentations and discussions that occurred during the workshop.

Chapter 2 reviews some of the statistics on health disparities and describes the four major determinants of health defined in *Healthy People 2010*: access to care, environment, genetics, and behavior. Chapter 3 includes Guyer's presentation of the paper, "A Systematic Literature Review and Economic Analysis of Intervention in the Preschool Period," describing the costs and consequences of interventions available to improve the health of children from birth to age 5, including the prenatal and preconception periods. Four areas of preschool child health were reviewed including tobacco exposure, obesity, injury, and mental health.

Bruner presented a paper he coauthored with Edward Schor of the Commonwealth Fund, entitled "Clinical Practice and Community Building: Addressing Racial Disparities in Healthy Child Development." The paper calls for a broad focus on total healthy child development, leading not only to improved child clinical health outcomes, but also improved outcomes including education, social development, and justice.

Chapter 4 discusses how the implementation of health policy can not only have far-reaching effects beyond the health of an individual child, touching the overall well-being of families and communities, but also how health policy can go beyond health, influencing education, economic welfare, and other aspects of a child's life. Ferguson spoke about the practical issues of implementing health policy and provided data from several successful policy programs. Sanders-Butler discussed the innovative health initiative that she has implemented in her school. "Healthy Kids, Smart Kids" supports academics and fights childhood obesity by giving students the information they need to be empowered to make healthy decisions.

Chapter 5 highlights three community-based approaches that are making a difference at both the local and national levels and that serve as examples of how individuals and communities can improve the health and lives of children. Johnson spoke about the Whitefoord Community Program she helped to found, which empowers residents of the Whitefoord Elementary School area to improve the health and education of their children. Kreuter and two of his colleagues who are community health workers, Roddie Longino and Travie Leslie, described their Atlanta-based initiative entitled "Accountable Communities: Healthy Together (ACHT)." ACHT is a community-based, participatory research effort funded by the National Center on Minority Health and Health Disparities. Giles provided an update on the progress of the "Racial and Ethnic Approaches to Community Health" (REACH) program. REACH communities are working toward bridging gaps between the health care system and the community; changing their social and physical environments to overcome barriers to good health; implementing strategies that fit their unique social, political, economic and cultural circumstances; and moving beyond individuals to community- and systems-level change. The open discussion that followed focused on budget issues and sustainability.

In Chapter 6, representatives from the business sector discussed their interests and investments in health and the role of business in improving communities and children's lives. White presented the perspective of a major health plan, WellPoint, Inc., an independent Blue Cross/Blue Shield licensee serving Georgia. Courton Brown also discussed a company's role in improving health in two different communities, the internal community that is the employees, and the external communities where the employees live and where the company does business. Kelly described ING's initiative to combat childhood obesity by sponsoring school-based running programs. Courton Brown and Kelly both provided perspective on why a non-health care company would invest in health.

Chapter 7 includes final comments from members of the Roundtable and the workshop audience. Discussion focused on sustainability of interventions, the link between spirituality and health, education of the next generation of physicians, and need for a social movement to bring everyone together and address health disparities nationally. Workshop chair Nicole Lurie provided closing comments.

Further information is provided in several appendixes. In addition to the meeting agenda (Appendix A) and biographical information about the speakers (Appendix B), websites for a number of the resources and model interventions discussed throughout the workshop are included in Appendix C, and the discussion of the video presentation *Unnatural Causes* is included in Appendix D. Appendix E is Bruner and Schor's commissioned paper.

2

Disparities in Children's Health: Major Challenges and Opportunities

D r. David Satcher, in his keynote address, described how investments in children's health can affect their later lives. In discussing the Healthy People 2010 initiative, he noted the four major determinants of health: Access to care, environment, genetics, and behavior.

Despite annual progress reports, it is still difficult to definitively say how far we have come toward the goal of eliminating disparities in health, said David Satcher, 16th U.S. surgeon general and director of the Satcher Health Leadership Institute at Morehouse School of Medicine in Atlanta, Georgia. He cited the IOM report, *Unequal Treatment: Confronting Racial and Ethnic Disparities in Health Care* (IOM, 2003) as a landmark in terms of increasing awareness about disparities in health and health care in the United States, and he noted that many efforts to address disparities have been undertaken by government, the private sector, and foundations across the country. Within the federal government, the Agency for Healthcare Research and Quality (AHRQ) issues a biennial report, the Health Services Research Administration (HRSA) has programs dealing with access to and quality of care, and the Centers for Disease Control and Prevention (CDC) supports the Racial and Ethnic Approaches to Community Health (REACH) program.

Many good community programs have also been established. Major health plans such as Aetna, Kaiser, and United have instituted programs dealing with disparities in health. Although these programs focus primarily on the quality of health care, insurers are also beginning to invest in communities to foster health. So while it may not yet be possible to measure the effects, the ongoing efforts are encouraging. The bad news, Satcher said, is that the programs have not been adequately supported. This is especially true for government initiatives such as those at the National Institutes of Health (NIH) and the CDC. As long as those programs are not adequately supported, he said, we cannot be fully confident that we are collecting all of the quality data that we need. The World Health Organization (WHO) believes that health inequities in the world can be eliminated in the next generation. The country in the best position to lead, Satcher said, is the United States. We have the resources and the constitutional backing, and we can lead the world by starting with our own country, but we need support and commitment.

Two of the overarching goals of *Healthy People 2010* are to increase years and quality of life and to eliminate racial and ethnic health disparities, although Satcher noted that it will take a few more decades beyond 2010 to fully realize these goals. Satcher concurred with Maupin that children's health is the most important investment we can make. Infant mortality is one of the most dramatic examples of disparities in health. African American babies are nearly two and half times as likely to die in their first year of life, and American Indian babies almost twice as likely to die, as the majority population. Interestingly, the United States trails other countries such as Cuba and Costa Rica in this regard, who although they have fewer resources than the United States, have lower overall infant mortality rates. Because we have failed to seriously make a commitment to eliminate disparities in health, we have pulled our whole health system down, and will continue to do so, Satcher said.

Worldwide, mortality of children under 5 years of age is about 80 per 1,000 live births. In the United States the rate is about 8 per 1,000 live births. Sweden has the lowest rate on record of about 3 babies per thousand who die before their 5th birthday. Sub-Saharan Africa, however, has an under-5 mortality rate of 172 per 1,000. The world cannot be stable and exist in peace, Satcher said, as long as such health inequities exist.

A study done at the Graham Center in Washington, DC, modeled what could have happened in the United States if disparities in health had been eliminated in the last century, assessing mortality ratios for African Americans and whites back to 1960 (Satcher et al., 2005). In 1900, the life expectancy in the United States was 47 years (49 for whites and 44 for blacks). Analysis of the data suggests that if disparities in health had been eliminated in the United States by the year 2000, there would have been 83,500 fewer deaths among African Americans. If infant mortality had been equal between both populations, 4,700 African American infants who died in the year 2000 would not have died. In terms of insurance coverage, there would have been 2.5 million fewer blacks uninsured, including over 600,000 children. In reality, in the year 2000 there were around 39 million people uninsured in this country, and in 2008 the number had increased to around 47 million.

Healthy People 2010 defined four major determinants of health: access to care, environment, genetics, and behavior. Figure 2-1 illustrates the interactions that take place among these various determinants of health. Environment and behavior have a tremendous effect on health. Our challenge, said Satcher, is to address the disparities associated with each of the determinants of health and to do it in an interactive fashion.

Environmental quality is a concern for African American and Hispanic children, who are much more likely to be exposed to toxic waste sites than other children. Twenty-five percent of preventable illnesses worldwide are caused by poor environmental quality. Mental health is also very important. The Office of the Surgeon General released a report in 2001 on disparities in the burden of mental illness as it relates to culture, race, and ethnicity (HHS, 2001a). The report concluded that there are tremendous disparities in the burden of mental illness owing to the lack of access to mental health services and the stigma associated with mental illness. For example, 1 in

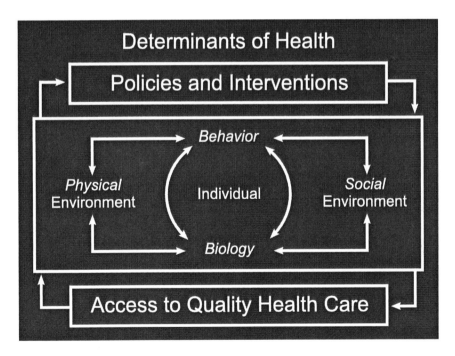

FIGURE 2-1 Determinants of health.
SOURCE: HHS, 2000.

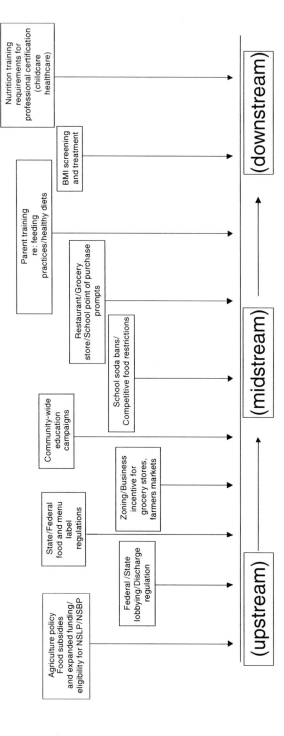

FIGURE 2-2 Population model of health promotion.
SOURCE: McKinlay, 1995.

10 American children and adolescents suffers from mental illness severe enough to cause some level of impairment, and fewer than 1 in 5 receives treatment.

Family violence also affects children, often resulting in injuries and death. Another report from the surgeon general concluded that youth violence is pervasive, and while certain racial and ethnic groups may be more likely to be arrested and sent to prison, youth violence is not limited to minorities (HHS, 2001b). The report concluded that intervention strategies exist that can be tailored to the needs of youth at every stage of development, and that there are programs that are effective in preventing serious youth violence.

Another example of an issue where intervention strategies are needed is childhood obesity, and obesity in general in the United States. The surgeon general's report on overweight and obesity details the dramatic increase in childhood obesity and the effect it has upon children (HHS, 2001c). One intervention, the Action for Healthy Kids program, engages schools in dealing with the obesity epidemic by helping them model good nutrition and increase students' physical activity. Schools now realize that there is a connection between learning and wellness. To be successful, Satcher said, we must attack the issues downstream, dealing with individuals and families, midstream in terms of community, and upstream, with policy initiatives. Figure 2-2 illustrates this concept of a population model for health promotion as it relates to healthy diets for children.

Satcher concluded by emphasizing that if we are to be successful in eliminating disparities in health we must first and foremost care enough. We also must know enough; research is critical and must continue at every level including the community-based research. Finally, we must be willing to do enough, and we must persist in our efforts.

REFERENCES

HHS (U.S. Department of Health and Human Services). 2000. Healthy people 2010: Understanding and improving health, 2nd ed. Washington, DC: U.S. Government Printing Office.

HHS. 2001a. Mental health: Culture, race, and ethnicity—A supplement to mental health: A report of the surgeon general. Rockville, MD: Substance Abuse and Mental Health Services Administration, Center for Mental Health Services.

HHS. 2001b. Youth violence: A report of the surgeon general. Washington, DC: Department of Health and Human Services.

HHS. 2001c. The surgeon general's call to action to prevent and decrease overweight and obesity. Washington, DC: Department of Health and Human Services.

IOM (Institute of Medicine). 2003. Unequal treatment: Confronting racial and ethnic disparities in health care. Washington, DC: The National Academies Press.

McKinlay, J. B. 1995. The new public health approach to improving physical activity and autonomy in older populations. In *Preparation for aging*, edited by E. Heikkinen. New York: Plenum Press. Pp. 87-103.

Satcher, D., G. E. Fryer, Jr., J. McCann, A. Troutman, S. H. Woolf, and G. Rust. 2005. What if we were equal?: A comparison of the black-white mortality gap in 1960 and 2000. *Health Affairs* 24:459-464.

3

Investing in Children's Health

In the presentations of their two review papers, Guyer and Bruner discussed the long term effects of early childhood interventions and their effects on later health and healthy child development.

Bernard Guyer of the Johns Hopkins Bloomberg School of Public Health presented the paper, "A Systematic Literature Review and Economic Analysis of Intervention in the Preschool Period," describing the costs and consequences of interventions available to improve the health of children from birth to age 5, including the prenatal and preconception periods (Guyer et al., 2008). The Partnership for America's Economic Success, which commissioned the Guyer review, comprises policy makers and business people who have come together to promote early investment in children as a strategy for improved economic success in the United States.

Charles Bruner of the Child and Family Policy Center presented a paper he coauthored with Edward Schor of the Commonwealth Fund entitled "Clinical Practice and Community Building: Addressing Racial Disparities in Healthy Child Development" (Bruner and Schor, 2008) (see Appendix E). The paper describes how clinicians need to focus on total healthy child development, not just the absence of disease. This broad focus affects child clinical health outcomes as well as other healthy development outcomes including education, social development, and justice.

INVESTMENTS TO PROMOTE CHILDREN'S HEALTH: A SYSTEMATIC LITERATURE REVIEW AND ECONOMIC ANALYSIS OF INTERVENTIONS IN THE PRESCHOOL PERIOD

Children are our future! Guyer began with a familiar quote, but for many who have worked in children's health for a long time, he said, this statement is at best, an overused cliché, and at worst, disingenuous. In fact, the level of actual government investment in young children in the United States has declined, and projections through the year 2017 based on current federal outlays predict a further decline of between 14 and 29 percent in investment in children's programs, the largest of which are the educational programs (Steuerle et al., 2007). The IOM report, *From Neurons to Neighborhoods*, emphasized the importance of infant brain development for future development and learning (IOM, 2000). Guyer and colleagues are working to build a parallel argument for the importance of investing in early childhood health, emphasizing the need to integrate a health focus into early childhood development and education.

Child health is more than simply the absence of disease and involves more than just providing access to medical care. Health is integrally linked to development and learning, and what happens in early life has implications across the life span. In addition, child health goes beyond the behavioral health of individual children. Child health is shaped by multiple determinants including social, environmental, economic, and genetic influences. Investing in early childhood health and development is a community responsibility and a communal investment.

Study Objectives and Approach

To help build this argument, Guyer and colleagues conducted a systematic literature review of both the short- and long-term effects of interventions in children from birth to 5 years of age, including the prenatal period and the period leading up to the pregnancy. Four areas of preschool child health were selected for study, including tobacco exposure, obesity, unintentional injury, and mental health, in part because they were highlighted in the *Healthy People 2010* and *2000* reports. The primary objective of the review, which covers literature from 1996 to 2007, is to assess both health and cost consequences in the four focus areas across the entire life span. The group focused particularly on economic studies that reported on either cost implications or cost-benefits of interventions. While the team sought randomized clinical trials first, in many cases they have not been done, and well-designed studies, using other kinds of evaluation designs that estimate economic costs, were therefore also assessed.

Data from the literature review were adapted to a framework that provides a life-course perspective. Interventions and effects from preconception and pregnancy through the preschool and childhood period and adolescence were assessed, as well as the effects of early intervention on health in adulthood (interventions in adolescence and adulthood were not assessed). The team looked at the level of intervention, meaning where the interventions took place: at the individual level, such as those delivered through a physician; at the family level; in communities, workplaces, or schools; or national or state policy-based interventions.

Tobacco

There is significant evidence of the link between exposure to tobacco in various settings and adverse health outcomes for young children. Over 10 percent of newborns have prenatal tobacco exposure, which is known to result in low birth weight and other pregnancy outcome complications. Twenty-five to 50 percent of American children are exposed to high levels of environmental tobacco, and teen smoking is a serious concern. The additional costs related to prenatal care and complications of birth that are attributable to maternal smoking amount to approximately $4 billion per year.[1] Direct medical costs of pediatric illnesses that are related to parental smoking reach nearly $8 billion per year. Estimates predict that a 15 percent reduction in parental smoking could net a savings of $1 billion per year in direct medical costs.

The evidence on tobacco is the most clear as it has been studied for the longest period of time, and there are good interventions with sound study designs presented in the literature. Interventions were identified at all levels, and there was evidence of cost reductions and cost implications across the entire life span (Table 3-1).

Obesity

The literature shows that among preschoolers, obesity has tripled in the last 20 years, increasing from 5 to 14 percent. More adolescents than ever are obese as well, with 17 to 18 percent of children ages 6 through 18 characterized as overweight. Fifty to 80 percent of overweight children and teens become obese adults with the potential for serious chronic health problems such as type 2 diabetes and cardiovascular disease. The economic impact of obesity is estimated to be $109 billion per year in direct costs, and $75 billion per year in indirect costs. The amount attributable to increased obesity-related hospitalizations for children aged 6 through 17 years increased four-fold between 1979 and 1999, from $44 million annu-

---

[1] All costs in this presentation were standardized to 2006 dollars.

TABLE 3-1 Examples of Reviewed Interventions

Child Health Areas	Intervention Levels			
	Individual	Family	Community/neighborhood	Society/policy
Tobacco exposure	Smoking cessation intervention for pregnant women	Smoking cessation for pregnant women with partner support; smoking cessation for adults living with children	Bans/restrictions in workplaces and public	Increasing the price of tobacco products and enforcing age bans
Obesity	Exercise program; dietary and physical activity; reducing TV watching	Obesity prevention education home visits	Healthier food served in preschools	
Unintentional injury		Prenatal home visitation; home visits that assess risks and provide education	Community education combined with giving incentives for road safety; primary-care-based education; smoke detector distribution	Changes in baby walker safety standards; child passenger safety laws
Mental health	Child-focused skills training; parenting skills training programs	Parent- and child-interaction training programs; collaborative parent problem solving; supportive consultation programs	Preschool-based programs including academic tutoring and teacher training	Employer-based work support through extensive child care assistance and health care subsidies

ally to $160 million. Guyer noted that it is very difficult to estimate the overall cost of obesity because these costs have not been followed throughout the entire life span.

Far fewer studies are available for obesity than for tobacco (Table 3-1). Guyer and colleagues did not find any studies that met their criteria for interventions in the preconception or pregnancy period that would address obesity during pregnancy, even though it is now known that obesity during pregnancy is associated with low birth weight and poor pregnancy outcomes. There were several small studies of preschool interventions and parental interventions, but no national or state policy studies on obesity were available at the time of the literature review (although the Robert Wood Johnson Foundation, Nemours Foundation, CDC, and others are discussing studies in this area).

Injuries

The third focus area was injuries, which are the leading cause of childhood death, hospitalization, disability, and emergency room visits. Fortunately, there have been some very successful interventions leading to a substantial reduction in injury mortality and morbidity rates in the United States over the last several decades. Reductions in unintentional injuries are the result of interventions such as good environmental engineering, better emergency medical services, and public health education fostering safer behaviors. The framework in Table 3-1 shows the range of interventions. This is the kind of integrated systematic approach that is needed in all of the focus areas, Guyer said. He noted that even though we have employed interventions such as bicycle helmets, gun safety, or home visits, the United States is still not investing at the levels needed to fully address childhood injuries.

Mental Health

The final area of review was mental health in the preschool period (children between the ages of 1 and 6). It is estimated that around 20 percent of children have at least mild mental functional impairments. For children between 1 and 6 years old, around 3 to 6 percent exhibit externalizing behaviors, and around 3 to 6 percent have internalizing behaviors. (The review did not include specific diseases, such as autism.) As shown in Table 3-1, there was an array of interventions. Most were clinically based interventions and small intervention studies, with very few done at the systems level. The available cost data was limited, but the estimated cost of treating children aged 1 through 5 years nationwide approached $864 million annually. The argument for better interventions early on to improve mental health for mothers and young children is something that clearly needs to be developed further, Guyer said.

Conclusions

Health problems of early childhood are antecedent to many of the health disparities and chronic diseases of adulthood. Health and economic consequences are high when followed across the entire life span. There is a body of evidence emerging that shows that something can be done about these problems by intervening early. Programs have been developed but have not been brought up to full scale, and systems are lacking. Effective programs and policies must be based on broad public health approaches, rather than relying on individual control or medical interventions alone. There are multiple societal determinants, necessitating multifaceted approaches, and there is a societal cost of failing to intervene.

As discussed earlier, much research has been done regarding tobacco exposure, and there is a great deal of ongoing research into childhood obesity. But mental health is an area that needs greater focus, and injury prevention is an area where advances have been made in the past, but renewed attention is needed. Guyer noted that literature on the effect of interventions early in life relative to reducing health disparities is also lacking.

More high-quality intervention studies are needed to demonstrate long-term effects and to convince policy makers to direct resources toward the early period of life. This is a "societal investment," promoting early childhood health both for the sake of the child and for the sake of promoting the health of the entire population.

CLINICAL PRACTICE AND COMMUNITY BUILDING: ADDRESSING RACIAL DISPARITIES IN HEALTHY CHILD DEVELOPMENT

How can we make well-child pediatric practice address all of children's needs for healthy development, Bruner asked, and what specifically around clinical health care practice can be done that also leads to community building? How do we address the determinants of good health that require nonmedical interventions, such as exposure to lead paint and other toxins?

Common Factors and Consequences

There are common factors that lead to racial and ethnic disparities in health: family factors such as poverty or stress; environmental factors such as safety or exposure to toxic substances; social factors including racism; and service factors including access, use, and quality of services such as clinical health services. All of these factors affect health outcomes, but, Bruner pointed out, they also affect education, social, and justice system outcomes. Together, they present a confluence of risk factors that produce a confluence of very poor child outcomes. The good news is that clinical health services are not alone in trying to affect all of these factors. To the extent we can affect child health, we can also affect other outcomes. But the clinical health services community does need to change its practice to be broader and to recognize that it has a partnering role with other institutions and organizations.

Figure 3-1 compares white non-Hispanic, black non-Hispanic, and Hispanic populations in terms of various selected health outcomes, health service access, education outcomes, and several other outcomes and conditions. For example, the percentage of children aged 6 to 11 years who are overweight is nearly double for black non-Hispanic children, and more than double among Hispanic children, compared to white non-Hispanic children. Some of the health disparities relate to the lack of a regular source of health care. Incomplete immunization rates in minority populations are also a concern. Lack of 4th-grade reading proficiency, 8th-grade math proficiency, and high school dropout rates are more than double in these minority communities. Other outcomes, for example, the incidence of 20- to 24-year-old males in prison, is significantly higher for African Americans.

	White NH	Black NH	Hispanic
Health Outcomes			
Low Birth Weight	7.2%	13.4%	*6.8%*
Elevated Blood Lead Levels (0-5)	2.6%	4.3%	3.1%
6-11 Overweight	11.8%	19.2%	<u>23.7%</u>
Health Service Access			
Lack of Regular Source of Care	3.3%	5.8%	**24.1%**
Incomplete Immunizations (19-35 mo)	16.7%	25.5%	21.3%
Education Outcomes			
Below Basic 4th Grade Reading	22%	<u>54%</u>	<u>50%</u>
Below Basic 8th Grade Math	18%	<u>53%</u>	<u>45%</u>
Non-completion of High School	21.4%	<u>48.8%</u>	46.8%
Other Outcomes			
Foster Care / 1,000	4.9	<u>15.8</u>	6.5
(20-24 year-olds) Male Prison / 1,000	9.5	**63.4**	<u>24.9</u>
Conditions			
Children in Poverty	11%	36%	29%
Children in Single Parent Families	23%	<u>65%</u>	36%
Pop. in High Vulnerability Tracts	1.7%	**20.3%**	**25.3%**

KEY:

Italics: lower than White, non-Hispanic

<u>Underlined:</u> more than 2x rate for White, non-Hispanic

Bolded: more than 5x rate for White, non-Hispanic

FIGURE 3-1 Comparison of selected disparities.
SOURCE: Bruner and Schor, 2008.

These are young men who may need to assume parenting roles for young children. The rate of children living in single-parent families is three times higher in the African American community. Clearly, serious disparities in health co-occur with other disparities around education, social development, and justice system involvement.

The Role of Clinical Practice in Addressing Disparities

Child health care practitioners cannot fulfill their role in child health without addressing more than clinical health conditions, Bruner said. They must focus on total healthy child development, which is not just the absence of disease. This broader approach affects clinical health outcomes, but it also affects other health and development outcomes including education, social development, and justice.

Figure 3-2 highlights some of the outcomes sought in well-child care for birth through age 5, related to physical health and development, child emotional, social and cognitive development, and family capacity and functioning. These are consistent with the most recent American Academy of Pediatrics (AAP) Bright Futures Guidelines, which provide a comprehensive and broad view of what a clinical practice can accomplish (Hagan et al., 2008). Not all of these are the responsibility of the clinical practitioner, but practitioners can contribute significantly to these outcomes through anticipatory guidance. For example, patterns of eating and exercise begin very young. The USDA's Women, Infants, and Children (WIC) nutrition program does a very good job educating those that receive WIC assistance about the importance of good nutritional habits. But there are still baby bottles filled with soda or juice because many parents simply don't know enough about good nutrition. The health practitioner can be that point of change.

At the family level, parents need to be knowledgeable about a child's physical health status and needs, and clinicians need to be alert to any warning signs of child abuse and neglect. But the health practitioner can also identify maternal depression, stress, and family violence. Although clinicians can't address all of these issues alone, they are a point of contact, and they need to help ensure support is provided.

The Importance and Prevalence of Place

Bruner and his staff at the Child and Family Policy Center conducted an analysis of all 65,000 census tracts in the United States and ranked them by the prevalence of 10 select factors related to "child vulnerability" such as single parents, poor families, aged 25 or older without high school completion, head of household on public assistance, and other similar situations. They then ranked the census tracts by the number of risk factors each had.

Outcomes of Well-Child Care During the First Five Years of Life	
Domain of Well-Child Care	**Outcome at School Entry**
Child Physical Health and Development	• All vision problems detected and corrected optimally • All hearing problems detected and managed • Management plans in place for all chronic health problems • Immunization complete for age • All congenital anomalies/birth defects detected • All lead poisoning detected • *All children free from exposure to tobacco smoke* • *Good nutritional habits and no obesity; attained appropriate growth and good health* • *All dental caries treated* • *Live and travel in physically safe environments*
Child Emotional, Social, and Cognitive Development	• All developmental delays recognized and treated (emotional, social, cognitive, communication) • *Child has good self-esteem* • *Child recognizes relationship between letters and sounds* • *Child has adaptive skills and positive social behaviors with peers and adults*
Family Capacity and Functioning	• Parents knowledgeable about child's physical health status and needs • Warning signs of child abuse and neglect detected • Parents feel valued and supported as their child's primary caregiver and function in partnership with the child health care provider • Maternal depression, family violence, and family substance abuse detected and referral initiated • Parents understand and are able to fully use well-child care services • *Parents read regularly to the child* • *Parents knowledgeable and skilled to anticipate and meet a child's developmental needs* • *Parents have access to consistent sources of emotional support* • *Parents linked to all appropriate community services*

Note: regular font bullets are those outcomes for which child healthcare providers should be <u>held accountable</u> for achieving. *Italicized bullets* are those outcomes to which child health care providers should <u>contribute</u> by educating parents, identifying potential strengths and problems and making appropriate referrals, but for which they are not independently responsible.

FIGURE 3-2 Outcomes of well-child care.
SOURCE: Bruner and Schor, 2008.

Those with six or more vulnerability factors have child vulnerability rates at two and half to nine times the level of others on these 10 indicators (Figure 3-3). Imagine, Bruner said, living in a community with no vulnerability factors, where half of America lives, versus living where there are six or more vulnerability factors, where opportunities, resources, and support are limited or not available.

When the neighborhood census tracts are broken down by race and ethnicity (see Figure 3-4), that data show that 83 percent of those with no vulnerability factors are white. Around 83 percent of those with six or more vulnerability factors are nonwhite. Of all white non-Hispanics, 1.7 percent live in census tracks with six or more vulnerability factors, compared with 20 percent all blacks and 25 percent of all Hispanics. About 7 percent of the white population and 50 percent of the Hispanic and the black populations live in communities with three or more vulnerability factors. If we do not have interventions and strategies that are focused on and appropriate to these neighborhoods where the children of color are living, Bruner said, we are not going to be able to affect those health disparities. Place has an independent effect on health outcomes. Environmental factors, family circumstances, and access to health services are factors, but it is also that this is the place where the children are, so how do we develop strategies that work in these neighborhoods?

	No Vulnerability Factors	Six or More Vulnerability Factors
% Single Parents	20%	53%
% Poor Families with Children	7%	41%
% 25+ No HS Completion	13%	48%
% 25+ BA or Higher	27%	7%
% HoH on Public Assistance	5%	25%
% HoH with Wage Income	81%	69%
% HoH with Savings, Dividend Income	42%	11%
% Owner-Occupied Housing	71%	29%
% 18+ Limited English	2%	18%
% 16-19 not School/Work	3%	15%

FIGURE 3-3 Child-raising vulnerability factors, 2000 Census data.
NOTE: BA = bachelor degree; HoH = head of household; HS = high school.
SOURCE: Bruner, 2007.

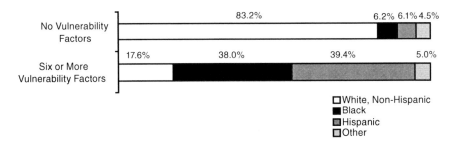

FIGURE 3-4 The importance/prevalence of place and race: Racial composition of census tracts by child-raising vulnerability, 2000 census data.
SOURCE: Bruner, 2007.

Help Me Grow: A Model for Clinical Practice

Bruner described the "Help Me Grow" initiative, a publicly funded program of the state of Connecticut Children's Trust Fund (Dworkin et al., 2006). It provides comprehensive well-child assessments and effective referrals to both clinical and nonclinical services. The program has strengthened and integrated community resources and has helped identify specific gaps in services. A primary component of Help Me Grow is physician education and training of health care providers in developmental surveillance, providing guidance on what screening should be done during well-child visits and how to elicit feedback from parents. Providers can refer parents, confident that there will be effective follow-up, as telephone care coordinators then contact the family to schedule the recommended appointments. Community health liaisons in the field identify resources and support that are available in the community and facilitate coordination (see Figure 3-5).

Bruner emphasized that the role of clinical practice in reducing health disparities extends beyond strictly medical interventions. As shown in Figure 3-5, some of the referrals are to programs under part C of the Infants and Toddlers with Disabilities Act (IDEA) or to professional clinical mental health services. But data from the model program shows that about one quarter of the issues identified for referral relate to parenting stress, lack of knowledge about child development, challenging child behaviors, and discipline issues around which parents feel a lack of control. Correspondingly, about one quarter of their referrals and actual scheduling of appointments relate to community-based parent support groups, church-related activities, community-based parenting education classes, and interventions that reduce the isolation and separation that parents often experience. There is clearly a role that pediatric practitioners can play in reaching out beyond strictly medical issues.

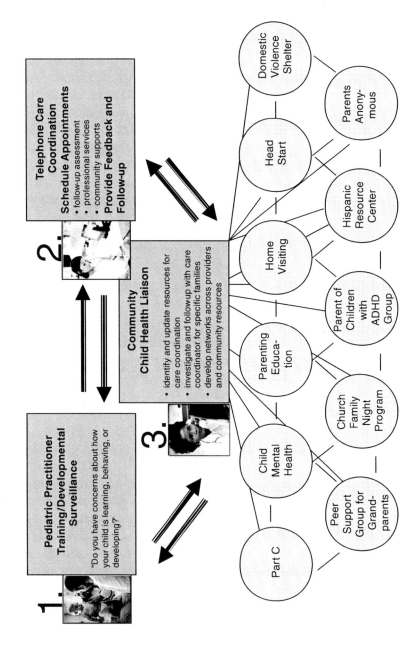

FIGURE 3-5 A model for clinical practice: Help Me Grow in Hartford, Connecticut.
SOURCE: Bruner and Schor, 2008.

Implications for Practice and Research

We don't have all the answers, Bruner said, but we do know enough to take action. There are some promising programs in place, but there needs to be diffusion of innovative strategies and incentives for moving these activities from exemplary programs to routine practice, including fiscal incentives, technical assistance, and recognition. Methodological rigor must be applied in assessing effects both around clinical child health, and then more broadly, in healthy child development. Randomized controlled trials are appropriate for some aspects of this work but are not applicable when assessing the success of building social support systems within the community.

The clinical health community needs to keep its focus on the clinical practitioner's role. Although there is a need for community development, for poverty reduction, and for a whole array of policies necessary to improve child health, these are not factors that the health practitioner can always control. A child health practitioner should not try to fill all the roles of child development specialist, family therapist, community resource, or community organizer. The health practitioner must provide the necessary clinical resources and use clinical expertise wisely. But it is not enough to simply advocate for others to intensify their own community-building efforts. There must also be changes within clinical practice. Bright Futures is an excellent model for a starting point. Practitioners need stronger links to community resources and can offer additional insight into resource needs for healthy child development. We need to know what preventive strategies work, Bruner said, for example what obesity prevention approaches are effective in the early years, or what types of practices can further reduce tobacco exposure through anticipatory guidance. The current research base on preventive primary pediatric practice is quite limited compared to the available research base on other clinical practices.

OPEN DISCUSSION

The open discussion that followed the presentation of the papers focused primarily on tobacco exposure. Bruner remarked that from a reimbursement perspective, smoking cessation programs should be covered by health insurance and Medicaid and ought to be actively promoted. He also noted the need for research demonstration programs on effective ways to limit children's exposure to tobacco smoke, as well as for encouraging parents to ensure a smoke-free environment for their children (e.g., by not smoking around their children or by quitting altogether). Satcher said restrictions on smoking in public places results in more people quitting smoking. Nicole Lurie commented that there is evidence from around the country that the tobacco industry has been targeting cigarette marketing at young black women with promotions such as two-for-one sales in their communities. She noted that this needs to be further investigated and addressed from a community perspective.

REFERENCES

Bruner, C., and E. Schor. 2008. *Clinical practice and community building: Addressing racial disparities in healthy child development*. Working paper. Des Moines, IA: National Center for Service Integration.

Bruner, C., M. S. Wright, and S. N. Tirmizi. 2007. *Village building and school readiness: Closing opportunity gaps in a diverse society*. Resource brief. Des Moines, IA: State Early Childhood Policy Technical Assistance Network.

Dworkin, P., J. Bogin, M. Carey, and L. Honigfeld. 2006. *How to develop a statewide system to link families with community resources: A manual based on Connecticut's "Help Me Grow" initiative*. http://www.commonwealthfund.org/publications/publications_show.htm?doc_id=462069 (accessed January 5, 2009).

Guyer, B., S. Ma, H. Grason, K. Frick, D. Perry, A. Wigton, and J. McIntosh. 2008. *Investments to promote children's health: A systematic literature review and economic analysis of interventions in the preschool period*. http://www.partnershipforsuccess.org/uploads/20081118_HopkinsPaperFINAL.pdf (accessed January 5, 2009).

Hagan, J. F., Jr., J. S. Shaw, and P. Duncan, Eds. 2008. *Bright Futures guidelines for health supervision of infants, children, and adolescents* (3rd ed). Elk Grove Village, IL: American Academy of Pediatrics.

IOM (Institute of Medicine). 2000. *From neurons to neighborhoods: The science of early childhood development*. Washington, DC: National Academy Press.

Steuerle, C. E., G. Reynolds, and A. Carasso. 2007. *Investing in children*. http://www.partnershipforsuccess.org/uploads/200801_UrbanPaperFINAL.pdf (accessed January 5, 2009).

4

From Policy to Practice: How Policy Changes Can Affect Children's Lives

This set of presentations describes some of the practical issues affecting the implementation of policies designed to have a positive impact on child health. The first presentation focuses on policies at the state level, while the second describes a program at the local level.

The implementation of health policy can have far-reaching effects, beyond the health of an individual child stretching to the overall well-being of families and communities, and beyond health, to education, economic welfare, and other aspects of a child's life. Christine Ferguson of the George Washington University spoke about the practical issues of implementing health policy and provided data from several successful programs. Yvonne Sanders-Butler of Browns Mill Elementary and Magnet School for High Achievers discussed the innovative health initiatives she has implemented in her school.

CHANGING HEALTH POLICY, IMPACTING LIVES

"There is no question, from my perspective, that policy intervention has an impact on outcomes," said Ferguson, who went on to cite several examples. A study by Szilagyi et al. (2006) followed a group of new enrollees in the State Children's Health Insurance Program (SCHIP) in New York State. Upon initial interview, 11 percent had a recent asthma-related hospitalization. One year later, the asthma-related hospitalization rate of the same group was 3 percent. While most would agree that this is a positive health outcome, it has other potential implications, such as a parent missing less work, or the child being absent less from school, and other effects on the family that one might not ordinarily consider. Obviously, the asthma-related hospitalization data does not prove that quality of life is improved. But, Ferguson said, in the absence of that specific data, we need to be able to make some inferences from the health data. It is clear that when you intervene and provide health coverage, there are better outcomes. Another study showed that children's average school performance also increased within the year after enrolling in SCHIP as measured by ability to pay attention in class and to keep up with assignments (Managed Risk Medical Insurance Board, 2002). More of this type of data is needed, Ferguson said, to aid the policy-making process and to help make the case that health care interventions have a very wide-ranging impact on a child's life.

Another study found that areas with greater Medicaid coverage experienced lower rates of preventable hospitalizations for children than areas with less Medicaid coverage. Children covered by Medicaid or SCHIP were equally as likely as children covered by private insurance to have had one or more visits to the doctor or health professional in the previous year, while uninsured children were 25 percent less likely. And approximately 3 percent of children with Medicaid/SCHIP delayed seeking medical care due to costs, only slightly higher than the 2 percent of children in private insurance. In comparison, 17 percent of uninsured children delayed medical care due to cost (Ku et al., 2007).

A fourth study Ferguson highlighted showed that children who had private insurance for either part of or the full year had about one more visit to the doctor each year than did uninsured children. Medicaid eligibility increased the probability of having at least one physician visit each year by about 10 percent. Compared to uninsured children, children covered with private insurance have more primary care visits, more preventive care visits, and more sick care visits each year; these visits translate into statistically significant improvements in immunization rates and an increased percentage of children screened for anemia, lead, and hearing and vision problems (Buchmueller et al., 2005).

Rhode Island RIte Care

From a commonsense perspective, Ferguson said, one of the best ways to ensure that pregnant women on Medicaid receive good prenatal care is to make sure that they have the same level of access to obstetrical/gynecological (OB/GYN) services that privately insured women have. This type of access was one of the quality improvements that were built into RIte Care, the Medicaid managed care program in Rhode Island implemented in the early 1990s, during the time Ferguson led the Department of Human Services (DHS) there.

Within a year and a half of implementation of the RIte Care program in

Rhode Island, the interbirth interval for women with low incomes became nearly the same as that of women with middle incomes (taking the source of insurance as a proxy for income) (Griffin, 2002). From a health perspective, the significant decrease in the percent of women on Medicaid with short interbirth intervals (less than 18 months between deliveries) is a positive health outcome. But beyond that, delaying having the second child can also mean the family is better equipped economically to support the growing family as a whole, so there is the potential for a positive effect on income-support programs. There is also likely a positive effect on education costs since families that have children with short interbirth intervals are more likely to access special education programs, Ferguson noted.

As part of the original proposal to the Centers for Medicare and Medicaid Services (CMS, which was the Health Care Finance Administration, HCFA, at the time), Ferguson said she requested that CMS require Rhode Island DHS to conduct a study on the impact and health outcomes of RIte Care on children and their families. Because such a study was then required by the agency, Ferguson had the justification to spend the money to do the research. Otherwise, it may not have been done.

New England has many very old houses, and another example of a policy intervention involves lead paint, known to cause numerous ill effects in children, including learning disabilities. One of the primary sources of lead in the home is the dust created when windows in casings painted with lead paint are raised and lowered. Many of the low-income housing landlords either are not willing or lack the money to invest in replacing all of the windows in a house. So it was decided that when a child was identified as having elevated lead levels, Rhode Island DHS would use Medicaid dollars to replace the windows and to conduct lead abatement in the house where the child lived. This program, unfortunately, was eliminated by CMS when the new administration came in. But the novel use of health care dollars in a way that supplements or supports the education system (by reducing lead-related learning disabilities), and the demonstration of how those health and education outcomes are linked, was very important. Ferguson noted that it is hard to sustain those kinds of interventions because we can't show what the impact is on the schools, or other parts of the system, in terms of making those investments.

Challenges

A particular challenge at the state government level in Rhode Island is that the state budget must be balanced at the end of the year, and it becomes a question of trade-offs and long-term versus short-term goals. Savings that result from an intervention must be demonstrated, and return on investment needs to be shown in the same year the investment is made, which is very unlikely, Ferguson said. One difficulty with health care and education initiatives is that the investments don't necessarily accrue rewards to the people who make the decisions to invest. A leader makes an investment and has perhaps eight years in office to see it through. Some programs can accrue returns within eight years, but others might not accrue for another 10 years.

In the research world, data can confirm that something has been a good investment. But administrators often have to overcome barriers of prejudice or bias when implementing new programs. That, Ferguson said, is why we still have disparities. Fundamentally, underneath all of the data and information are a series of deeply held core beliefs that trump data. And what we do not do well is either figure out how to present the data in a way that appeals to the bias (because it may be morally reprehensible to so many of us) or find a way to change perceptions about the fundamental bias. As researchers, we tend to think that the data are so clear, it should speak for itself. That is a significant challenge going forward.

Next Steps

Ferguson offered several suggestions for going forward. Using smoking as an example, she noted that we have to be more clear what the effect of an intervention is on other people, whether it is an economic effect or a personal effect. With smoking, of course, the tipping point was the data showing how smoking in public places affected other people.

We have to be willing to take risks in how we use data, and we have to have some sympathy for those who are trying to apply the data in policy development. We must understand the need to spin data in a particular direction to get the job done. We need ways to connect the policy makers, decision makers, and leaders with the researchers, and we need people who can translate between the two groups. We need to provide leaders with support when they inevitably come up against resistance because they are pushing the envelope on a sensitive issue. We must enable leaders to take risks and to allow some of these difficult conversations to take place.

We need to do a better job of creating networks. We need to keep key people rotating through different leadership roles. For example, a school principal who institutes change may at some point be relieved by the school board who thinks he or she has pushed too far. The same thing happens with state government leaders; so shifting those people around, and putting them in different roles exposes new people to their ideas.

HEALTHY KIDS, SMART KIDS

Although many people call her "the sugar-free school principal," Yvonne Sanders-Butler introduces herself as a "survivor" of childhood and adult obesity. She has firsthand experience about children, nutrition, and how nutrition affects learning, behavior, and socialization. The causes of obesity start at a very young age, and for Sanders-Butler, her habits and addictions with food started as early as 3 years old. She almost lost her life to a stroke in the mid-1990s, the result of a lifetime of overeating, eating foods that were very poor in nutrition or had little or no nutritional value, and leading a high-stress life. For 20 years or more, she had been dieting, was 50 pounds overweight, had become prediabetic, and became one of 60 million people who suffered from the diseases that were brought on by obesity, hypertension, high cholesterol, and depression. She had to make a behavioral change as prescribed by her physician to live. This was very difficult after 30 years of poor eating habits and little or no exercise, but her research proved she was not alone. She joined a 12-step support group and for the first time realized she was addicted to certain foods that triggered certain behaviors. The support from her family, friends, and colleagues helped her to make a major, life-saving lifestyle change.

As an educator and an elementary school principal, she saw that the children in her school were following the same pattern she had as an adolescent and adult. However, her children were on a fast track, with high levels of fast-food consumption and little and or no exercise. Many of these children could well lose their lives in their early 30s or late 20s due to obesity-related illnesses.

With children, Sanders-Butler said, you have to deal with parents, and she didn't know quite how to tell them but she believed only brutal honesty would get their attention—and it did. She informed parents that if they did not make a change in their children's nutrition and in their physical activity, they would bury their children at a very young age. She shared with them research showing that this is the first generation of children who would die before their parents die.

Sanders-Butler's school, Browns Mill Elementary, is in the most affluent area of DeKalb County, Georgia. Parents influence school administration and not vice versa. But she felt she was brought to her school to make a difference, and before students can be educated, they have to be healthy. The pivotal moment for Sanders-Butler was one day when she was on lunchroom duty and observed a young overweight boy trading the last of his baseball card collection to another student for chocolate milk and fudge cookies. It was that day, she said, that she decided to create the first sugar-free school in the United States. This was the beginning of Browns Mill School's wellness policy.

Sanders-Butler met with the parents of the Browns Mill Elementary students and shared with them that test scores were less than ideal, and although this was an affluent geographic area, their children were not performing any better than children attending Title 1 schools in impoverished communities. To get the parents' attention, she compared schools and academics. The parents were eager to remedy the situation, but were less enthusiastic when Sanders-Butler proposed that the solution was a change to their diet, removing high-sugar, high-calorie foods. She emphasized that the 130 first graders, if they continued on the path they were on with poor diets and no physical activity, would probably be not only overweight and obese, but they would be hypertensive, and some could even have strokes as early as 18 to 22 years old.

Finally garnering the parents' support, she moved to get the students to buy into the program, knowing that they would be the ones who would actually sell the approach at home. The program, entitled "Healthy Kids, Smart Kids," supports academics and fights childhood obesity by giving students the information they need to know about their health so that they will be empowered to make healthy decisions (Sanders-Butler, 2005). She enlisted the students' support by identifying the student leaders and making them a part of the program.

Although sugar was the primary focus, overall Browns Mill implemented healthier menus. They removed at least 85 percent of the processed sugar from the menu and also looked for items that were baked and not fried, and items that were lower in salt. For students who bring lunch from home, there is a preferred snack list, and parents have adopted the diet because children can only bring certain foods to school. Sanders-Butler visited 15 grocery stores in the community to ask them to provide foods that would support the families in meeting the goals of the program. Before the program began, there were many 5-year-olds coming into kindergarten already overweight. Now their younger siblings are starting school, and they have been on the same diet at home and are not overweight. The local churches where many students attend are also supportive.

In the first year of implementing this program, discipline concerns dropped 28 percent. Sanders-Butler used to see a large number of students in her office for disciplinary issues immediately after breakfast, which used to include items such as pancakes with syrup and chocolate milk. But the real test, she said, was when the school saw a 15 percent gain in math and reading scores in the state-mandated standardized tests.

When Sanders-Butler entered Browns Mill 10 years prior, 23 percent of students received free and reduced-price lunch. Research shows that when a school is largely filled with reduced-price lunch recipients, their standardized scores are correspondingly low. Demographic shifts in DeKalb County show that Browns Mill is now at 50 percent free and reduced-price lunch,[1] yet test scores are higher than ever before, confirming that nutrition and physical activity are connected to not only the health of students but to how they perform.

Unfortunately, it was apparent early on that there was no funding available for what Sanders-Butler set out to do. So she convinced her husband to mortgage their home, which was almost paid off. The funds were used to partly help assess the school environment, bring in subject matter experts such as nutritionists and fitness experts to provide staff training, help plan school initiatives and projects, and help plan activities for the school and the community. Outside experts also provided advice on how to create and implement a schoolwide curriculum across content areas. Finally, the funds were used to purchase a variety of vegetables, fruits, and beverages that were not offered in the school cafeteria. An investment she fully believed in has clearly paid off. There are 102 elementary schools in the district, and Browns Mill is the most requested school in DeKalb County. People move to the area because of the Healthy Kids, Smart Kids program. We have some very good data now, Sanders-Butler said. The school has been named a Georgia School of Excellence twice and was also named a National Blue Ribbon School. This would not have been possible had there not been an environment created that fostered excellence.

DISCUSSION

In the discussion following the two presentations, one attendee asked whether the Browns Mill program changed diets in the students' homes or in the broader community. Sanders-Butler noted that two-thirds of a child's nutritional needs can be provided in the school setting, which is critical given the increase in students eligible for free and reduced-price lunch. She also worked with grocery stores to ensure that the appropriate foods were available to students and their families. Ferguson stated that schools also need to talk about what schools themselves can do to support families.

Another participant asked if there was a role for community organizations in getting school districts to change their nutritional and physical activity policies. Ferguson noted that what is critical is identifying a couple of people in key leadership roles who are willing to take a risk and connecting them with policy leaders.

A Morehouse College student commented that eating healthy is expensive for a starving college student, and that it is easier and cheaper to eat

---

[1] Although considered an affluent community, Sanders-Butler said, after 9/11 people were losing jobs at an alarming rate, and the economy has continued its downturn over the last 7 years, resulting in the increased need for subsidized meals.

unhealthy choices. Sanders-Butler said that buying food in bulk helps to not only reduce costs but allows for the preparation of several meals over a period of time. Although fast-food might appear to be less expensive, it is only eaten for one meal. The notion that healthy foods are more expensive is not necessarily true if one thinks about what it costs over time to eat unhealthy choices.

REFERENCES

Buchmueller, T. C., K. Grumbach, R. Kronick, and J. G. Kahn. 2005. The effect of insurance on medical care utilization and implications for insurance expansion: A review of the literature. *Medical Care Research and Review* 62:3-30.

Griffin, J. F. 2002. The impact of RIte Care on adequacy of prenatal care and the health of newborns: 2000 update. Barrington, RI: MCH Evaluation, Inc.

Ku, L., M. Lin, and M. Broaddus. 2007. Improving children's health: A chartbook about the roles of Medicaid and SCHIP. http://www.cbpp.org/schip-chartbook.pdf (accessed January 12, 2009).

Managed Risk Medical Insurance Board, California Department of Health Services. 2002. Health status assessment report: First year report. Sacramento, CA: California Department of Health Services.

Sanders-Butler, Y., and B. Alpert. 2005. *Healthy Kids, Smart Kids: The principal-created, parent-tested, kid-approved nutrition plan for sound bodies and strong minds.* New York: Perigee Books.

Szilagyi, P. G., A. W. Dick, J. D. Klein, L. P. Shone, J. Zwanziger, A. Bajorska, and H. L. Yoos. 2006. Improved asthma care after enrollment in the state children's health insurance program in New York. *Pediatrics* 117(2):486-496.

5

Community Development Approaches: Overcoming Challenges, Striving for Change

Although many communities have initiated programs designed to reduce health disparities, a single community will want to address problems and solutions that are unique to them. At the same time, however, there are common ideas and elements to these programs across communities. This chapter highlights three community-based approaches that are making a difference at both the local and national levels, serving as examples of how individuals and communities can improve the health and lives of children. Veda Johnson of Emory University spoke about the Whitefoord Community Program she helped to found, which empowers residents of the Whitefoord Elementary School area to improve the health and education of their children. Marshall Kreuter of Georgia State University and two of his colleagues who are community health workers, Roddie Longino and Travie Leslie, described their Atlanta-based initiative entitled "Accountable Communities: Healthy Together." Wayne Giles of the Division of Adult and Community Health at the Centers for Disease Control and Prevention (CDC) provided an update on the progress of the Racial and Ethnic Approaches to Community Health (REACH) program.

WHITEFOORD COMMUNITY PROGRAM: CARING FOR CHILDREN IN THE CONTEXT OF FAMILY, HOME, AND COMMUNITY

Health disparities are multifactorial, Johnson said, and she prefers to approach children's health in a very holistic manner, going into the community and caring for them in the context of everything that affects their lives.

In 1994, Johnson and the late George Grimley (also of Emory University) decided that to better care for children, the two had to go where the children were. Health disparities were not a focus at the time. Rather, access to health care was the primary issue they were trying to address. They set up the Whitefoord Elementary School-Based Center, located in Southeast Atlanta, as a typical practice with pediatric primary health services for the children who attended the school and their preschool siblings. Johnson and Grimley's goal was to increase access to quality health care and thereby improve the academic achievement of the students.

Initially, students came to the clinic when they were sick, and they were treated accordingly. But after 2 or 3 months Johnson discovered that physical health really was not the greatest issue facing the children, and that their health outcomes were not entirely contingent upon whether their ear infection was treated or their asthma was controlled. Instead, the outcomes for children were centered on psychosocial, academic, and family issues. She then saw the clinic as an entry point for interactions with the families. Out of the clinic grew the Whitefoord Community Program, a community-based, community-driven organization designed to care for children in the context of everything that affects their lives, their family, their home, and their community. The program empowers residents to take charge of themselves, their children, and their community.

Community Needs

The Whitefoord Community Program is based on the needs that were identified by the families in the community. Johnson noted that it is very important to go into the community and ask questions. Sometimes there is a tendency to think we know what families, communities, and individuals need, when in fact we really do not. You need to go out and live among people to really begin to understand what their challenges are, and why they do what they do, she said.

Based on the discussions, it was clear that the mission of the program would be greater than just direct medical intervention; in fact, the mission evolved to a focus on working with families in the community to ensure that every child had the ability to succeed in school. The primary need identified was increased access to quality health care to address chronic health problems such as asthma, diabetes, and obesity in the community, as well as issues of youth violence, teen pregnancy, substance abuse, and mental health disorders. The families also wanted more affordable, high-quality early childhood education and after-school programs. Some parents said they needed adult literacy and General Educational Development (GED) instruction so that they could better teach and mentor their own children. (Prior to initiation of the program, about 50 percent of the families did not have a parent with a high school diploma.) Families also needed more direct social services in the community, including parenting support, and more importantly, counseling for the parents so they could better deal with the stresses in their own lives and thereby be better able to manage the lives of their children.

Planning and Implementation

As discussed above, the first step in planning the program was working with the community to identify and prioritize needs. The next step was to collaborate with everyone in the community who had a role in caring for children—schools, parents, community leaders, community agencies, and potential funders—to develop programs to address each of the needs. An advisory committee was established within the schools to monitor and evaluate the effectiveness of the programs. Finally, community members were recruited to be on the board of directors to participate in governance of the organization.

The Whitefoord Community Program is run out of a series of five homes across the street from the Whitefoord Elementary School, where the first school-based health center was established. There are three major components of the program: school-based clinics, of which there are now two; a child development program that currently cares for about 75 children; and a family learning and community development center that provides GED instruction for families, and after-school programs, summer programs, and mentoring programs for children.

Services and Staffing

The in-school clinics are comprehensive and holistic. Clinic services include management of acute and chronic illnesses and injuries; routine and sports physicals; immunizations; dental care; mental health assessments and counseling, including services for adults; psychoeducational assessments and testing to identify children who are at risk for failing; and referrals to medical specialists and social services.

The clinics are staffed by medical providers, including physicians, nurse practitioners, physicians assistants, nursing assistants, a dentist and dental assistant, social workers, and mental health providers. There is also a full-time health educator, as health promotion and disease prevention is the best approach to decreasing health disparities, and administrative staff.

Funding

Funding for the Whitefoord Community Program comes from a variety of sources. Medicaid alone, Johnson noted, is not sufficient. Neither are reimbursements from private insurers. Currently, 35 to 50 percent of the funding for the center comes from a Health Resources and Services Administration (HRSA) federal grant. Medicaid and private reimbursement supply about 25 percent of the funding, philanthropy about 20 percent, and in-kind donations (e.g., clinic space, utilities, malpractice insurance) make up about 5 to 10 percent.

Programwide Accomplishments and Individual Success Stories

The Whitefoord Community Program has some impressive programwide accomplishments. Overall, the program has increased community access to quality medical and dental care. Over 5,000 children have received medical care since the program began in 1995. The clinics are currently the medical home to about 1,000 children, but in reality, the clinics see about 1,500 to 1,600 children and adults per year. There is very strong support from the schools and community, with 95 percent clinic enrollment and utilization. Johnson believes that this speaks to the quality of their approach to caring for children. The immunization rate for 2-year-olds is about 90–92 percent. The immunization rate for adolescents in the same families is also high, at 82 percent.

School attendance has improved, especially among children who have chronic diseases such as asthma. Johnson believes that performance has also been positively affected, but improvement has not yet been measured directly. Every child in the school receives health education on drug and substance abuse, violence prevention, safety, general health, and nutrition. The program goes into the classrooms and provides about 8,000 student health education encounters every year.

Children with chronic illnesses, especially asthma, have shown improved health outcomes. Eight percent of the asthma visits to the clinic are children who are asymptomatic, a result of the very aggressive approach to managing these children. The program also improved the health outcomes for the children who are overweight. Since an after-school fitness and nutrition program was implemented several years ago, about 50 percent of the children have had a reduction in their body mass index (BMI), and 40 to 50 percent of the children have had a decrease in their cholesterol level and fasting insulin level.

A very important accomplishment, Johnson said, is the increased parental involvement. The program has been able to impart to them the importance of having an active role in the lives of their children, and families are engaged even when it is difficult or stressful for them. There has also been a reduced cost to the state's Medicaid program and decreased emergency room use and hospitalization of students with asthma (Adams and Johnson, 2000).

As important as these program-based figures are, Johnson likes to measure success one child and one family at a time. Among the examples she cited were the ability to detect a brain tumor in a third-grader while it was in the early stage and treatable, the early detection of a genitourinary deformity in a 9-year-old child that was successfully corrected, and early detection and intervention of children with chronic illnesses such as asthma and diabetes.

In addition, through onsite counseling and support, the program has facilitated the recovery of many emotionally troubled children. This, Johnson noted, is probably the most important aspect of the program as far as improving the outcomes for children. Unless you adjust the emotional aspect of the health of people, she said, you will not be able to make improvements in their physical health.

In meeting needs and bridging gaps, Johnson concluded, the program has been able to increase access to health care, improve health outcomes for children and their families, decrease health care costs, and improve school attendance and academic performance.

ACCOUNTABLE COMMUNITIES: HEALTHY TOGETHER

Atlanta, Georgia is divided into 25 neighborhood planning units (NPU). The NPU system was established by Mayor Jackson in 1974 to ensure that citizens, particularly those who have been historically disenfranchised, would have a voice in the structure and development of their community. Accountable Communities: Healthy Together (ACHT) is a community-based, participatory research effort that Kreuter and colleagues are conducting in NPU-V (letter V). ACHT is funded by a grant from the National Center on Minority Health and Health Disparities (NCMHD), which supports a collaboration between the NPU-V community leadership and the Georgia State Institute of Public Health, the Centers for Black Women's Wellness, the Atlanta Regional Health Forum, the Fulton County Department of Health and Wellness, and the Southside Medical Center. The ACHT program, Kreuter explained, engages the community in identifying their health issues, providing them with the methods, activities, and data to do so, and then identifying pilot programs to take action on those health problems.

The neighborhood data advisory group (NDAG), composed of local residents, developed a profile of NPU-V in 2004. The NDAG identified an unambiguous pattern of health, social, and environmental disparities in

NPU-V. Examples include physical or mental disability at twice the citywide rate; high school graduation at half the citywide rate; infant mortality at two and a half times that of white infants; owner-occupied housing at half the citywide rate; overweight among women at 64.5 percent versus 44 percent among women citywide; male cancer mortality 50 percent higher than for white men in the state; diabetes prevalence 48 percent higher than a decade prior; 68 percent of households with incomes less than $25,000; and 25.4 percent of reported major crimes classified as violent versus 16.8 percent citywide.

As described in the IOM report *From Neurons to Neighborhoods*:

> It is important to emphasize that early biological risk and insults, such as iron deficiency, often do not occur in isolation. In fact, they typically are increased among infants who also grew up in a disadvantaged environment. . . . It can be exceedingly difficult to disentangle poor development and behavioral outcomes that are due to the biological exposure from those due to the problematic environment. (IOM, 2000, p. 206)

And in fact, Kreuter said, in NPU-V it is the environment that is the culprit.

Health Data Collection and Community Listening Sessions

NPU-V has about 16,000 residents, 94 percent of whom are African American, said Longino. As described above, the community is burdened by a disproportionate number of health, social, and economic disparities. After receiving the NCMHD grant for the community-based, participatory research program, community health workers were recruited and trained, and collection of health information for NPU-V began.

One primary source of health information was medical records from Southside Medical Center. Records were reviewed to determine the most frequent diagnoses for NPU-V residents who presented at the hospital. The data showed that the neighborhood mirrors the national pattern for disadvantaged populations, with hypertension, diabetes, asthma, and disorders of the skin, eyes, and teeth being the predominant complaints.

To help assess disparities, health indicators in NPU-V were compared with those in another Atlanta neighborhood, NPU-F. Demographic data from the year 2000 show that NPU-V was 90 percent black with 68 percent of homes having an income of less that $25,000, while NPU-F was 85 percent white with 40 percent of households earning more than $75,000. Despite the marked differences in race and income, the differences in vacant housing were less dramatic, with 88 percent of houses in NPU-V occupied, compared to 95 percent in NPU-F. However, by 2007, only 58 percent of the housing in NPU-V was occupied, with 42 percent of houses vacant.

Geographic information system (GIS) maps provided by the Georgia Department of Human Resources enabled the team to compare similar health problems in the two neighborhoods. Figures 5-1, 5-2, and 5-3 compare NPU-V and NPU-F with regard to the rates of all cancer deaths for males, type II diabetes prevalence for males, and type II diabetes prevalence for females, respectively. In all three examples, the rates are higher in NPU-V. But notice the pattern, Longino said, when the incidence of breast cancer in females is compared between the neighborhoods (Figure 5-4). The incidence of breast cancer in NPU-V appears lower. The different pattern was puzzling at first, Longino said, until it was determined that in this case, incidence reflects how many women were screened for breast cancer. The breast cancer mortality rate in females in NPU-V is 50 per 100,000, nearly twice that of NPU-F at 26 per 100,000. Clearly, low rates of screening correspond to higher rates of mortality. The question to be answered next is if this low rate of screening is due to lack of knowledge about the importance or availability of screening, lack of access or transportation to screening, lack of insurance, or a combination of all of these things.

Another phase of data collection was small group community listening sessions (about 15 to 20 people per group) employing "perception analyzer" technology. This approach is an effective alternative to focus groups. Each participant received a handheld device that he or she used to instantly and anonymously register his or her responses to questions. Everyone has an opportunity to respond, participants remain engaged throughout the presentation, and the tallied responses can be displayed in real time, spurring further discussion. Participants in the listening sessions, for example, were shown the GIS maps on breast cancer incidence and the data on mortality, described above, and were asked to provide instant feedback using the perception analyzer. Eighty percent of the participants indicated that they were not aware of the disparity.

As another example, residents were asked how many days during the previous month they would say their mental health had not been good. Twenty-six percent said that their mental health was not good for 14 days or more, which is considered to be "frequent mental distress." This is consistent with the national pattern of mental health findings in disadvantaged communities. By comparison, only 12 percent of residents in a statewide survey indicated mental distress 14 days or more within a month.

Social Determinants of Health

In addition to collecting health data, the team sought to understand the social and environmental determinants of health, starting with the loss

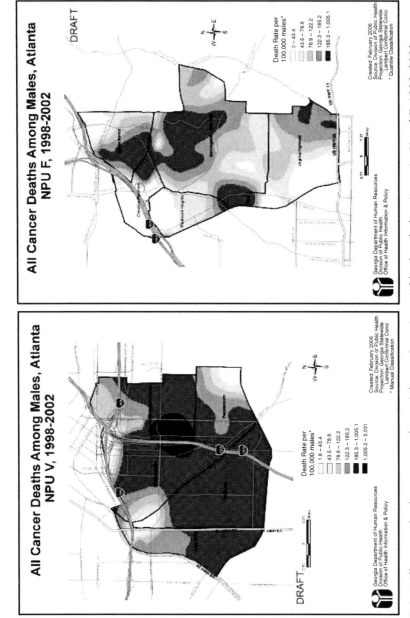

FIGURE 5-1 All cancer deaths among males in Atlanta, Georgia, neighborhood planning units V and F, 1998–2002.
SOURCE: Georgia Department of Human Resources Behavioral Risk Factor Surveillance System.

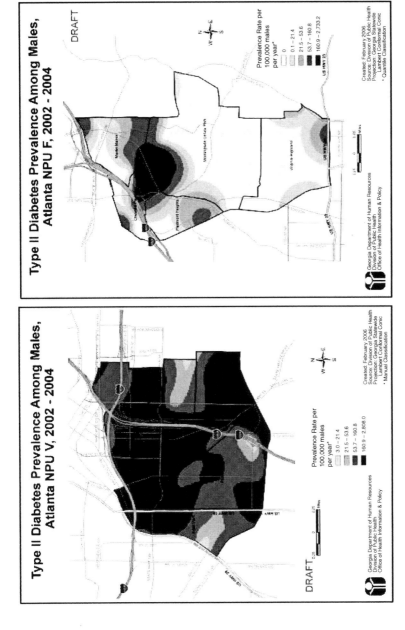

FIGURE 5-2 Type II diabetes prevalence among males in Atlanta, Georgia, neighborhood planning units V and F, 2002–2004. SOURCE: Georgia Department of Human Resources Behavioral Risk Factor Surveillance System.

44

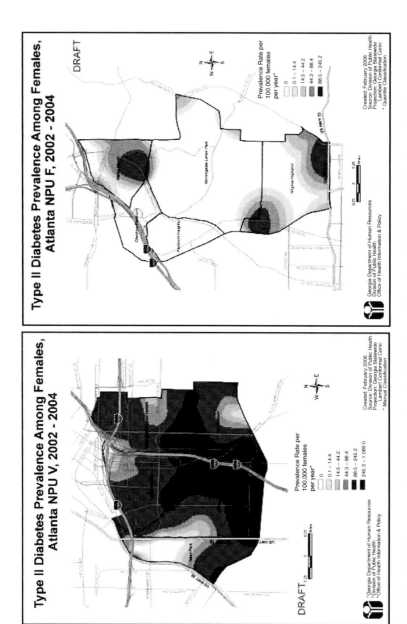

FIGURE 5-3 Type II diabetes prevalence among females in Atlanta, Georgia, neighborhood planning units V and F, 2002–2004.
SOURCE: Georgia Department of Human Resources Behavioral Risk Factor Surveillance System.

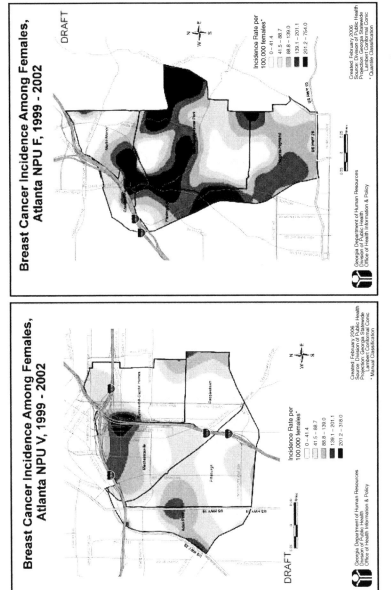

FIGURE 5-4 Breast cancer incidence among females in Atlanta, Georgia, neighborhood planning units V and F, 1999–2002. SOURCE: Georgia Department of Human Resources Behavioral Risk Factor Surveillance System.

of businesses in the community. The first half of the 1900s saw a steady increase in businesses in the community, peaking at 178 businesses in NPU-V by the early 1960s. But between 1964 and 2006, the community saw an 86 percent decline in the number of local businesses, with only 26 remaining in 2006. You don't have to be an economist, Leslie said, to understand that losing 80 percent of local businesses, and therefore also local jobs, is not good for community health.

To study the social environment, the team used "photovoice," a qualitative method that combines photography and grassroots social actions to better understand how residents see the conditions they live in, and to bring these graphic realities to the attention of policy makers. Leslie cited one photovoice submission from a 7th grader in NPU-V. Describing the picture she took of a boarded-up home, the girl said "This is an abandoned house with lots of trash. Anybody from criminals to rapists could just walk in and make themselves at home. I've been in the Pittsburgh community for a long time, and this house is one of the issues in our community. When I walk by this house on the way to school with my friends, it makes us worried, especially the little kids."

Another photovoice picture of a house in disrepair was used as part of a campaign entitled "The Dirty Truth." The campaign was designed to spread the message about the high number of vacant properties in NPU-V, and the associated concerns including increased crime, rodents and pests, pollution, strained community services, and poor physical and mental health. This campaign also enabled the documentation and update in the percentages of vacant properties from 12 percent vacant to 42 percent vacant.

Establishing Priorities and Pilot Interventions

In August 2006 a community meeting was held to set priorities for NPU-V based on the health and social environment information collected. Participants marked ballots with what they perceived to be the two most important local health issues and social determinants of health (Figure 5-5). Residents then voted a second time on a subset of items that received the most votes. The residents' first priority health issue was mental health and depression, and they saw this as a root cause of other problems. Interestingly, the data from the Southside Medical Center presented by Longino earlier did not list mental health as one of the top 10 diagnoses stemming from hospital visits. The reason, Leslie said, is because the hospital does not screen for it. But based on their experience, the residents identified depression and mental health as a top concern for NPU-V.

After establishing the priorities, the NCMHD grant required several pilot interventions be undertaken. The first intervention was improving access to mental health services through a clinic-based strategy designed

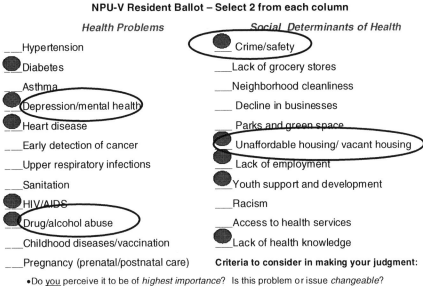

FIGURE 5-5 NPU-V resident ballot to establish community priorities.
SOURCE: Kreuter, Longino, and Leslie, 2008.

to improve the rates of follow-up support services. The second was the Dirty Truth campaign, mentioned above. Using the photovoice method as an advocacy and community empowerment strategy, the campaign was designed to improve the environment and housing problems (factors that are known to influence depression and hopelessness) through changes in local policies and enforcement practices. "Everyone Deserves to Work," the third pilot intervention, is an innovative strategy to reduce crime by providing social support and connection to services for reentry candidates (ex-offenders). It pairs previously incarcerated individuals, male and female, with a resident sponsor who is willing to help them navigate through the system of job placement, job training, and so on.

Finally, during the listening session there were repeated references to residents using the 911 system for health care. Analysis of emergency medical services (EMS) data at Grady Memorial Hospital led to a 2-year pilot grant funded by the Healthcare Georgia Foundation to determine whether a strategy to make primary care services more available to NPU-V residents would result in a decline of EMS and 911 services for nonemergency health needs.

Accomplishments and Challenges

Examples of accomplishments of the ACHT pilot interventions to date include demolition of several hazardous structures, increased access to mental health services at the Center for Black Women and Wellness, and as noted above, support from the Healthcare Georgia Foundation to address the nonemergency use of 911 and emergency services.

Challenges fall into two basic categories: community challenges and institutional (university) challenges. For the community, a key challenge has been developing trust. Other challenges include balancing differences in perspective, priorities, assumptions, values, beliefs, and language, determining who "speaks" for the community, and documenting intervention success. A significant challenge at the institutional level is institutional review board (IRB) approval of interventions. Recall that this is community-based participatory research. Other institutional challenges include time-consuming processes, budget issues, benefits for community health workers, documenting intervention success, and the inability to fully specify all aspects of research up front.

Leslie concluded with advice for those who undertake the community-based participatory approach, from her perspective as a community health worker and NPU-V resident. Remember that we are people, not subjects or experiments, she said. Also be aware that there is a "research disparity" in that the university gets all the indirect costs, which is not a "partnership" in the eyes of the community. Collaboration and trust are not one-time events—they are fragile and need constant care. The roles of social, racial, and economic determinants of health have been known for decades. Disparities cannot be resolved in 2, 5, or 10 years time, and funding support must reflect this reality.

RACIAL AND ETHNIC APPROACHES
TO COMMUNITY HEALTH (REACH)

"We must endeavor to eliminate, so far as possible, the problem elements that make a difference in health among people," Giles began, offering a quotation that could have easily been current, but in fact was written by W.E.B. Dubois over 100 years ago, in 1899, in the first systematic review of the health status of a non-Caucasian population in the United States.[1] We are still talking about those same disparities, Giles said, and while we do need to continue to document disparities, what we need now is action. We can't still be documenting these disparities 100 years from now.

The disparities are well known. Heart disease death rates are 30 percent

---

[1] W.E.B. Dubois, *The Philadelphia Negro*, 1899, p. 148.

higher for African Americans than whites, and stroke death rates are 41 percent higher. Diabetes is more prevalent among American Indians and Alaska Natives (2.3 times), African Americans (1.6 times), and Hispanics (1.5 times). Vietnamese American women have a higher cervical cancer rate than any other ethnic group (5 times non-Hispanic white women). African American infants are 2.5 times more likely to die before their first birthday.

Racial and Ethnic Approaches to Community Health (REACH) is a national program instituted by the CDC to eliminate racial and ethnic disparities in health by providing grants to support community-based interventions. Partners supporting the REACH program include the Office of Minority Health, the Office of the Assistant Secretary for Program Planning and Evaluation, the Administration on Aging at the Department of Health and Human Services, the Office of Minority Health and Health disparities at the National Institutes of Health (NIH), and the California Endowment.

REACH is about empowering community members to seek better health, Giles said. REACH communities are working toward bridging gaps between the health care system and the community; changing their social and physical environments to overcome barriers to good health; implementing strategies that fit their unique social, political, economic, and cultural circumstances; and moving beyond individuals to community- and systems-level change.

Health Disparities *Can* Be Overcome

The number one lesson learned, Giles said, is that disparities in health are not insurmountable and they can be overcome. In South Carolina, for example, there are REACH communities that are focused on diabetes among African American men and women. They have been able to reduce low-extremity amputations among African American men with diabetes by 36 percent and 44 percent in Charleston and Georgetown counties, respectively, over the last 8 years. These are people who otherwise would have been severely disabled from their diabetes. A second example, in Lawrence, Massachusetts, focused on Latinos with diabetes and has demonstrated a nearly 9 percent improvement in blood sugar levels, 18 percent improvement in systolic blood pressure, and 14 percent improvement in diastolic blood pressure.

A REACH community in Fulton County, Georgia, and others across the country, are conducting blood pressure and cholesterol screenings at the barber shop as young men are sitting down to get a haircut. The barber is trained to talk with them about physical activity and healthy eating. In Charlotte, North Carolina, a local farmer's market was established to provide access to affordable fresh fruits and vegetables, and as an added benefit, it also helps local farmers. Survey data indicate an increase in fresh fruit and vegetable consumption among African Americans in Charlotte.

Although these examples of community-specific results are encouraging, it is important to assess the program's impact nationwide. The REACH Risk Factor Survey compares data from all REACH communities with the larger U.S. population, and larger racial/ethnic subpopulations. A survey covering 2002–2006 shows that cholesterol screening for Hispanics living in REACH communities is increasing, even while nationwide fewer Hispanics are being screened. And within the REACH communities, cholesterol screening of African Americans is actually greater than the national average for all races.

Today, only one out of every three people with hypertension has their blood pressure adequately treated and controlled. Nationwide, although there has been an increase in the percentage of people with hypertension who are on medication, among American Indians nationwide there has been minimal change. However, among the REACH communities the number of American Indians with hypertension who are taking medication has increased.

Finally, cigarette smoking among Asian men has historically been very high compared to the rest of the nation. But in REACH communities, the percent of Asian men who smoke is now lower than the percentage of Americans of all races who smoke. Disparities are not insurmountable, Giles reiterated, and said we need to teach other communities how to do what these communities have done so well.

Why REACH Works

Echoing the comments of other speakers, Giles said there have been a number of challenges around community-based participatory research, including time; coordinating federal and community priorities; forming successful community, academic, and governmental partnerships; ownership; power; and division of resources.

First, community-driven programs and policy development are key, said Giles. During a planning year, the community developed an action plan, which was extremely important in terms of the success of the REACH program. This participatory activity led to the empowerment of individuals within the community to take charge of their own health. It also empowers the community as a whole. In the Bronx in New York City, for example, most people in the community were not aware that there were disparities in diabetes and cardiovascular disease. When they found out, they mobilized and traveled to Albany, New York, and talked with state policy makers about creating safe places for physical activity. In Los Angeles, California, members of a REACH community worked with the city council to establish a moratorium on new fast-food restaurants in south central Los Angeles. When you mobilize communities, Giles said, they are empowered to approach policy makers about these issues.

A second key component for success is having community, academic, and governmental partnerships. All of the REACH community coalitions were required to include a state or local health department, an academic or research institution, and a community-based organization. This has not necessarily been easy, Giles said, and many of the communities struggled with this. For example, when the academic institution wants to conduct a survey and publish the results, the community members also want to see the results and be part of the analysis and interpretation. During the planning phase of the study, residents had the opportunity to have this type of important dialogue, and it helped to move the process forward and helped the communities be more comfortable with the partnerships they engaged in.

Community expertise is very valuable. Given time and guidance, the community members are really best suited to determine the types of interventions that should occur in their community. In Charleston, South Carolina, community members developed a program called "Praisercize" where older residents do chair aerobics to gospel music. They have become local celebrities, and now they travel around the state to county fairs demonstrating Praisercize.

Finally, relying on the communities is an important aspect. This is a very different approach for CDC, and it has been challenging for the CDC staff conducting the community-based participatory approaches. But REACH has proven to be a successful partnership, and it has been exciting to watch how the communities have grown. REACH has been able to give communities a sense of hope. They have the tools and the sense that there is something that they can do to eliminate disparities. An example of this is the Golden Girls in Charleston, who go out walking in their neighborhood every day. The idea of creating safe places for physical activity is important, as is giving communities the tools to actually make changes.

REACH-ing Further

Communities need to be aware of and understand health disparities in their daily lives, Giles continued. They need to establish interventions, and then they need to teach other communities about what worked for them. To facilitate this, REACH funds 16 Centers of Excellence in the Elimination of Health Disparities (CEED). At the centers, regional and national experts serve as mentors for other communities. These experts offer information about how to address disparities, and the centers provide small seed grants to communities to begin the discussion around disparities elimination.

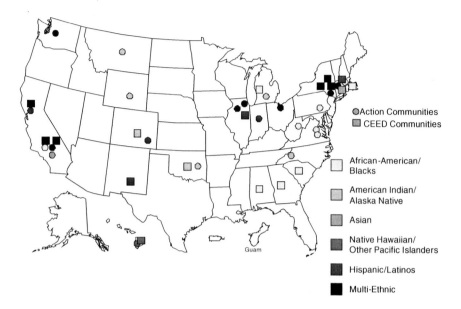

FIGURE 5-6 REACH communities in the United States.
SOURCE: CDC, 2007.

In addition to the centers of excellence, there are 22 action communities involved in the implementation and evaluation of established and innovative interventions (Figure 5-6).

Giles concluded by emphasizing that over the last 9 years, REACH communities have been able to show that disparities can be addressed and can be eliminated.

OPEN DISCUSSION

Much of the discussion that followed the presentations focused on budget issues and sustainability. We need to find creative ways to document the effectiveness of interventions, and we need to be much more politically active in terms of communicating effectively with legislatures, Kreuter said. Even programs such as SCHIP, which has demonstrated efficacy, was difficult to obtain funding for early on.

Leslie noted that as a community health worker, she has seen the disparities in her neighborhood, and said they are caused by the lack of essential services, the lack of interest from political leaders, and the lack of government identifying and providing what is needed in order to close the health gaps. Funding is badly needed, and she emphasized that the communities are not asking for a handout, but a hand up. Giles concurred with the funding issues. Kansas City, Missouri, he said, was one of the communities that REACH did not have the resources to continue to fund. Instead of discontinuing the interventions, the community mobilized and raised $400,000 to continue the work of the community. This is a real example of community empowerment and shows what can happen when the communities realize the value of what they can accomplish. But, Giles said, there does need to be more federal dollars for this type of work. There were over 200 communities applying for REACH, and CDC was only able to fund 40.

Johnson noted that there are two very important issues around sustainability. First, initial funders have unrealistic expectations that there will be results in 2 or 3 years. They need to be made to realize that this is a long-term generational approach to changing the health climate for families. Second, everyone is conducting similar work in different silos. We need to integrate and collaborate so we can use the paucity of funds more effectively, she said.

In response to a question about the costs of clinic services provided by the Whitefoord program, Johnson said that the clinics are federally qualified health centers (FQHCs), and there is a sliding fee scale, with some patients charged a zero fee. She noted that because hers is a school-based clinic, a large number of the children are seen without the parents being present. While the clinic does not follow up with the parents regarding the fee, it does make an attempt, when families come in together, to make them aware that the clinic is an FQHC, and that they are responsible for paying something.

REFERENCES

Adams, E. K., and V. Johnson. 2000. An elementary school-based health clinic: Can it reduce Medicaid costs? *Pediatrics* 105(4 Pt 1):780-788.

CDC (Centers for Disease Control and Prevention). 2007. *REACH-U.S. Grantee partners.* http://www.cdc.gov/reach_us.htm (accessed July 8, 2009).

IOM (Institute of Medicine). 2000. *From neurons to neighborhoods: The science of early childhood development.* Washington, DC: National Academy Press. P. 206.

6

Do Businesses Have a Role Improving Communities or Improving Children's Lives?

In this session of the workshop, representatives from the business sector discussed their interests and investments in health, and the role of business in improving communities and children's lives. Although it may not be intuitive that private businesses would be interested in child health, the presenters offered an important perspective on why non-healthcare companies might be interested in investing in child health.

Sandra White, medical director for WellPoint, Inc., presented the perspective of a major health plan. She described how WellPoint works to foster better health not only for the community composed of their plan members, but also for the community at large, and how they developed member and state health indices to track the success of health initiatives. Michele Courton Brown, senior vice president of charitable management services with Bank of America, also discussed a company's role in improving health in two different communities, the internal community that is the employees and the external communities where the employees live and where the company does business. Examples of children's health issues addressed by programs supported by the Bank of America include after-school care, exercise and nutrition, and oral health. Maureen Kelly, director of sponsorships at ING in the United States, described ING's initiative to combat childhood obesity by sponsoring school-based running programs. Courton Brown and Kelly both provided perspective on why a non-health care company would invest in health.

WELLPOINT, INC., BLUE CROSS/BLUE SHIELD

As an independent licensee of Blue Cross or Blue Cross/Blue Shield plans, WellPoint serves 35 million members across 14 states (California, Colorado, Connecticut, Georgia, Indiana, Kentucky, Maine, Missouri, Nevada, New Hampshire, New York, Ohio, Virginia, and Wisconsin). Well-Point provides a catalyst for planning, facilitating, and improving health care through support of the patient–physician relationship, aligning incentives to support patient quality outcomes, and designing benefit plans to meet consumer and employer needs. A variety of specialty medical services are provided through brands such as WellPoint NextRx, which manages pharmacy benefits, and WellPoint Behavioral Health. Lumenos provides consumer-driven health solutions; disease and integrated care management is provided through Health Management Corporation (HMC); HealthCore conducts health outcomes and health services research; and American Imaging Management (AIM) provides radiology management.

The mission of WellPoint, White said, is "to improve the lives of the people that we serve and the health of our communities." To measure success in meeting this mission, WellPoint launched two health indexes, the Member Health Index and the State Health Index. The Member Health Index monitors prevention and screening, case management, clinical outcomes, and patient safety of WellPoint plan members. The State Health Index provides a comprehensive look at the health of the population in the areas of maternity and prenatal care, preventive care, lifestyle, and morbidity and mortality. The State Health Index includes the entire population for that state, not just the members of a WellPoint health plan.

Measuring Success: The Member Health Index

The Member Health Index was created to measure WellPoint's success in its mission of improving the lives of the people it serves, those who are members of WellPoint health plans. Areas that have potential to affect the quality of care that members receive are assessed, such as product design, quality management, disease management, or provider contracting. Clinical areas included in the Member Health Index are grouped into four domains of health care services: screening and prevention, care management, clinical outcomes, and patient safety (Box 6-1). The index builds on information management capabilities and partnerships with employers, physicians, hospitals, and members. The index is reported as a single enterprise-wide number that reflects the overall care WellPoint members receive.

BOX 6-1
WellPoint Member Health Index:
Domains of Health Care and Clinical Areas

Screening and Prevention
- Breast cancer screening
- Cervical cancer screening
- Colorectal cancer screening
- Screening adults for high cholesterol
- Childhood immunizations

Care Management
- Diabetes compliance
- Hypertension compliance
- Rate of behavioral health follow-up within 7 days
- Long-term controller medication prescribed to asthmatics
- Appropriate treatment for upper-respiratory infection
- HMC disease management participation rate
- HMC-managed diabetic and CAD members with controlled blood pressure

Clinical Outcomes
- ED visits per 1,000 for short-term diabetes complications
- ED visits per 1,000 for congestive heart failure
- ED visits per 1,000 for uncontrolled asthma
- Hospital admissions per 1,000 for heart attack, stroke, and TIA ("prestroke")
- 30-day readmission rate for congestive heart failure, diabetes, and asthma

Patient Safety
- Patient Safety Hospital Structural Index (AHRQ safety measures)
- Patient Safety Outcome Index (LeapFrog safety measures)
- Annual monitoring of patients on persistent medications

NOTE: AHRQ, Agency for Healthcare Research and Quality; CAD, coronary artery disease; ED, emergency department; HMC, WellPoint Health Management Corporation.

Measuring Success: The State Health Index

The State Health Index tracks eight measures (chosen out of a total of 23 measures as established by CDC) of public health. These eight measures were selected for focused efforts to improve statewide outcomes, and to be the basis for measuring WellPoint's success in the 14 states where WellPoint holds a Blue Cross or Blue Cross/Blue Shield license: Prenatal care in the first trimester; low birth weight infant rate; adult influenza immunization rate; adult pneumococcal immunization rate; physical activity rate; cigarette smoking rate; diabetes in the adult population; and heart disease death rate. The WellPoint Foundation provides support for the State Health Index through the "Healthy Generations" initiative, which funds programs to improve the health across the lifespan. Healthy Generations is a multigenerational approach to improving public health and is focused on improving the measures included in the State Health Index.

White presented data from the host state, Georgia, to highlight why these eight particular measures were selected as focus areas of the State Health Index. With 1 being the best and 51 being the worst, Georgia ranks

- 33rd in the country for low birth weight,
- 26th for prenatal care in the first trimester,
- 46th for meeting recommended levels of physical activity,
- 34th for cigarette smoking rate,
- 44th for adult influenza immunization rate,
- 39th for adult pneumococcal immunization rate,
- 41st for diabetes in the adult population, and
- 39th for heart disease death rate.

Clearly, these areas require improvement, and WellPoint initiatives are focused on

- increasing the percentage of mothers in the state who engage in prenatal care during the first trimester of their pregnancy;
- the percentage of adults age 65 and over who receive influenza and pneumococcal vaccines;
- the percentage of the population meeting the CDC recommendation of at least 30 minutes of moderate physical activity 5 or more days a week, or at least 20 minutes of vigorous activity 3 or more days per week; and
- decreasing the percentage of newborns who weigh less than 5.5 pounds, the percentage of adults in the state who smoke cigarettes, the prevalence of adult diabetes, and the death rate from coronary artery disease.

With the exception of adult immunization rates for influenza and pneumococcal vaccines, all of the focus areas affect children's health. Box 6-2 highlights WellPoint State Health Index activities focused on children.

BOX 6-2
WellPoint State Health Index: Activities Focused on Children

Prenatal Care in the 1st Trimester and Low Birth Weight Infant Rate
(Colorado, Connecticut, Georgia, Kentucky, Missouri, Ohio, Virginia)
- Parent Partnership: Prenatal care for at-risk pregnant teens
- March of Dimes prematurity education and awareness campaigns
- Kentucky State Health Department and Western Kentucky University:
  Prenatal, primary care, and smoking cessation programs for pregnant
  women
- March of Dimes "Stop Smoking, Stop SIDS" program

Cigarette Smoking, Diabetes, Heart Disease
(Multistate programs and partnerships)
- Last Cigarette for Young Adults, ages 18–30
- American Heart Association "START!" program: Calls on Americans and
  employers to create a culture of health and physical activity for longer
  heart-healthy lives
- "Health MPowers" brings programs and technology into kindergarten
  through 8th-grade classrooms to promote healthy behaviors among
  students, faculty, and families

Compliance with CDC Recommended Levels of Physical Activity
(California, Colorado, Georgia, New Hampshire, New York, Ohio)
- Governor's Council on Physical Fitness "Live Like a Champion" program:
  City-to-city tour teaching elementary school children importance of eating
  healthy and outdoor physical activity
- "Fit4Colorado" and "America on the Move": Promotion of healthful eating
  and active living
- YMCA family fitness and "Granite State Fit Kids": Statewide teaching New
  Hampshire 5th graders about healthy eating and activity habits
- Adopt-a-School with New York Road Runners Foundation "Mighty Milers"
  program: Promotes physical activity in school-age children in the five
  boroughs of New York City
- Ohio Association of Free Health Clinics: Supports "Free to Be Healthy"
  project addressing obesity and related health problems

Another reason why these particular focus areas were selected, White said, was because of the rising costs associated with obesity, tobacco, sedentary lifestyle, and stress. Between 1987 and 2002, there was a 62 percent increase in private health insurance costs due to population risk factors and treatment of these particular conditions. An average 10 percent of total claims costs are attributable to obesity, with 60 percent of Americans exceeding the ideal body mass index (BMI) and 60 percent performing no substantial activity or exercise. Twenty-five percent of Americans smoke, and an average 10 percent of total claims costs are attributable to tobacco. Two-thirds of all office visits to family physicians are due to stress-related symptoms, and more than one in four workers has taken a day off to cope with stress, costing U.S. businesses $300 billion annually in direct and indirect costs.

The WellPoint Foundation

The WellPoint Foundation and the Blue Cross/Blue Shield of Georgia Foundation provide grants to nonprofit organizations whose efforts support the goals of the State Health Index. In 2007, the WellPoint Foundation granted $10.8 million to 76 organizations, and $23 million was pledged through the Annual Associate Giving Campaign to support 9,600 not-for-profit agencies. The Blue Cross Blue Shield of Georgia Foundation made $1.6 million in grants to 20 organizations. In addition to grants for programs, both organizations engage in social responsibility giving, for example, providing funding for adult flu and pneumonia vaccinations, or supporting the American Cancer Society's Relay for Life. WellPoint's social responsibility giving totaled $4.8 million with 76 percent supporting state health measures, healthy lifestyles, and major diseases. Blue Cross/Blue Shield gave $320,000, with 86 percent supporting these three areas.

The WellPoint Foundation has also committed $30 million over 3 years to reduce the number of uninsured through support of such organizations as the Foundation for Healthcare Coverage Education (FHCE). FHCE raises awareness of no-cost and low-cost coverage options, simplifies public and private health insurance information in easy-to-use pamphlets and an educational website (coverageforall.org), and operates the U.S. Uninsured Helpline, which provides information in several languages about federal and state programs. White noted that some of the uninsured have chosen to be so (in some cases because they are young and healthy and don't believe they need insurance), but many others are simply not well informed about what is available to them.

WellPoint Health Plan Programs: Reducing Disparities

WellPoint is a leader in working to eliminate health disparities among its members, White said. To help reduce health disparities, WellPoint provides cultural competency training for all clinical associates within the organization. In addition, WellPoint provides member materials translated into 12 different languages at a 6th-grade reading level. Member focus groups are used to identify behavioral drivers of disease and to develop culturally and linguistically sensitive member educational materials and disease management programs.

WellPoint also analyzes quality measures by race and ethnicity, which allows them to address health disparities at community levels, White said. By linking race and ethnicity data to geographic data, local "hotspots" can be identified. These hotspots can be used to focus WellPoint's interventions with regard to both location and approach, aiding the development of culturally sensitive programs. For example, using the ZIP code map laid out across the counties of Georgia, WellPoint identified areas where the mammography screening rates are lowest (Figure 6-1). Meshing that with information about the regions (e.g., rural or urban, racial breakdown) they can develop interventions, or provide materials and support to providers, in order to help them improve the screening rates. Analysis can be done at many different levels, including by provider group. By identifying the demographics of provider groups, WellPoint is able to work closely with

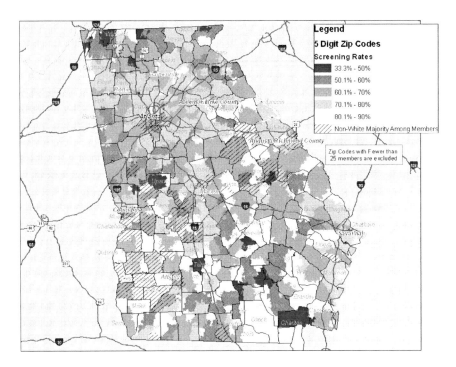

FIGURE 6-1 Mammography screening rates for Georgia, by ZIP code.
SOURCE: HHS, 2006.

those providers to ensure that they have the tools to help them serve their multicultural patient population.

In conclusion, White said that WellPoint is working to put all the pieces of the puzzle together to improve health, including foundation support (community giving, social responsibility, reducing the number of uninsured); health systems (physician quality, hospital quality, health information technology), community initiatives (collaboratives, public health programs, WellPoint State Health Index); and health plan programs (care management, disease management, disparities reduction programs, WellPoint Member Health Index).

BANK OF AMERICA

The business community has a significant role to play in the lives of the communities we work in, said Courton Brown, based on her experiences as a corporate donor and as an advisor to foundations. Businesses have long been engaged in the lives of their communities through employee work/life programs as well as through local community involvement.

The Employee Community

There are many ways in which companies can add value to their community of employees, both directly as employers and by providing opportunities for their employees to add value to the workplace. Some of the common work/life programs include flextime and part time, employee assistance programs, paid volunteer days, company matching charitable gifts, tuition reimbursement, and backup child care. These programs complement the suite of traditional health insurance and dental insurance programs offered by companies. There are also employee-led initiatives. At Bank of America, for example, a resource group focusing on issues affecting employees with disabilities held a number of workshops around the country on the issue of children with learning differences. This brought value to our employee population, Courton Brown said, helping our employees navigate the sometimes complex world of supporting children who have learning style differences.

Traditional Community Outreach

One of the primary attributes of a large company is the ability to provide financial resources, through grants or other programs, to help address social issues. But another treasured resource at the company, Courton Brown said, is the employees, who have both the propensity to give and the willingness to bring their individual talents and skills to the nonprofit community. Bank of America, like other companies, has a volunteer network. It also seeks to place its employees on the board of directors of nonprofit organizations, and offers in-kind support as well.

The corporate community serves a wide variety of constituencies beyond their primary customers. Other key corporate stakeholders include employees and the community, as well as good stewardship of the environment, human rights, and diversity. In the last 15 years, Courton Brown said, there has been a movement from simple corporate philanthropy to a focus on being a responsible corporate citizen. Companies are addressing the way in which they conduct business and supporting public policy changes to enhance communities. Companies have moved away from transactional "checkbook philanthropy," to more proactive, strategic, and outcome-oriented grant making, often in partnership with others in the community. In addition, the Internet provides round-the-clock news, which enhances transparency and helps keep companies accountable.

Investing in Health

There are many good reasons why a non-health care company, such as Bank of America, should focus on health, Courton Brown said. There is documented evidence that good health outcomes are linked to long-term productivity. Businesses understand that having a healthy community is helpful to their bottom line, whether it is developing the next generation of the workforce or making their work locations attractive to new employees. Prospective employees today are looking for healthy communities, and companies have a role to play in supporting community health, not only to sustain their workforce, but also to improve the quality of life in those communities. There is obviously a vested self-interest on behalf of the companies, which is a good thing, Courton Brown asserted.

Corporations are demonstrating their commitment to health care in a variety of ways. One example is the "After-school for All" partnership in Boston, Massachusetts. In 2001, a group of civic and business leaders came together to address the critical need for after-school care, a priority that had been articulated by Boston's mayor, Tom Menino. Boston, like many cities, has a school system that does a good job, but is stressed, Courton Brown said. Many middle schools in Boston run from 7 a.m. until 1 p.m. That gap between when school lets out and when parents arrive home from work presents a real challenge. Business community and civic leaders joined forces to make an initial $1 million commitment in support of after-school programming. Interestingly, the funders decided to make this a real learning opportunity, first conducting research to determine exactly where funding was needed. Bank of America, and other companies, chose to fund individual after-school programs, improving the quality and the number of after school slots in company hometowns, but there was also the opportunity to pool resources and fund some programs collectively. Ultimately, 130 organizations were funded through this program, with $26 million invested in after-school programming. Another task of the partnership was to find a way to sustain this program after the initial 5-year commitment. A new program called "Boston After-school and Beyond" is now in place that allows for streamlining of both city and private resources to continue the momentum on after-school care.

Another Boston-based program is "Jump Up and Go," which was initiated by Blue Cross/Blue Shield of Massachusetts. According to the 2001 Massachusetts Youth Risk Behavior Survey, one quarter of Massachusetts high school students were either overweight or at risk for becoming overweight. Inactivity and poor diet contributed significantly to this problem. Blue Cross/Blue Shield took the lead in this effort, helping organizations that serve youth, including community-based organizations, health care centers, and clinicians, to create a healthier environment for Boston's children. Among the key initiatives of the multidimensional Jump Up and Go program is the creation of the "5-2-1" campaign. The key messages are to eat five or more servings of fruits and vegetables a day, limit screen time for children to no more than 2 hours a day, and get at least 1 hour of physical activity each day. There has been a 5-2-1 media campaign, and clinicians now have a resource kit that supports their dialogue with patients about healthier lifestyles. Blue Cross/Blue Shield also initiated the Healthy Choices Program, which has engaged, to date, 55 percent of the state's middle schools, working with physical education and health teachers to create healthier school environments. One of the outputs has been a change in the vendor mix in the schools, replacing carbonated sodas with healthier beverages and adding more healthy food choices to school lunch programs.

The third example Courton Brown described was the "Watch Your Mouth" campaign, a private-public partnership focused on children's dental health. Tooth decay is a disease, and poor dental health affects children's performance in school. Watch Your Mouth helps educate families about the need for proper oral care and provides community resources to assist in obtaining preventive services, such as sealants.

Strategic Corporate Community Involvement

All of these strategic corporate alliances have several things in common. First, they leverage corporate expertise. The rigor that companies apply to the analysis of data is helpful in these kinds of projects. Second, these projects are public-private partnerships, and there is real value added to these programs because companies sought the expertise of practitioners to help shape the programs. Third, the funding community is becoming increasingly focused on outcomes, and the ability to measure outcomes is built into the programs. Finally, Courton Brown said, while it is great to have a good idea and execute a successful program, long-term sustainability is a common key goal.

ING FOUNDATION

Corporate sponsorships, Kelly said, are able to help draw attention to societal problems. The ING "Run for Something Better" program is helping ING to draw attention to the serious problem of childhood obesity. ING became involved initially through its sponsorship of marathons. Now the program provides funding for school- and community-based youth running programs across the country. The Run for Something Better program introduces kids to the benefits of running and encourages them to embrace physical fitness and healthy lifestyle choices.

The program in New York City maintains partnerships with the New York Roadrunner's Club and the Mighty Milers after-school program. With funding from ING, additional schools were able to be added to the program. ING also works with the city parks foundation in New York to support the city parks and recreation programs, allowing the program to continue year-round. In Miami, Florida, ING has created partnerships with the Fit Miami Foundation, the Miami-Dade County public schools, and a local company, PR Racing, which runs the Miami marathon. At the 2007 marathon, 1,700 children in orange ING T-shirts crossed the finish line as part of a 25-week program where children run 1 mile a week. Then on marathon weekend they run their last 1.2 miles on the final leg of the same course as the full marathon runners, completing a total of 26.2 miles, and everyone receives a medal. In Denver, Colorado, ING is the lead sponsor of "Kids Running America," a program similar in structure to the Miami marathon, with children completing their final mile at the Denver marathon. The inaugural ING Georgia marathon was held in March 2007, and ING launched a pilot program with the Atlanta Public School System, starting with four schools and now including close to 20 schools. In San Francisco, California, the ING "Bay to Breakers" is a 12k Race, in partnership with AEG, the Staples Center Foundation, and others, along with the San Francisco Unified School District. ING has offices in Hartford, Connecticut; Minneapolis, Minnesota; Minot, North Dakota; and Philadelphia, Pennsylvania, and will be expanding to include partnerships with the local schools in those communities.

Benefiting the Community and the Business

There are multiple reasons why ING developed this program. As a global financial services company, ING believes it has a responsibility to be an outstanding corporate citizen, especially in communities where its employees live and where it conducts business. Clearly, the childhood obesity statistics are startling, Kelly said, but the good news is that increased awareness is prompting teachers and parents, as well as communities, businesses, and concerned individuals, to step up and take action. ING's primary goal was, and continues to be, to increase public awareness of obesity and the associated health risks and to raise money to fund track and field programs for children in underserved schools and communities.

The race sponsorships also help ING establish itself in the community. In the corporate world, there has to be a business reason for taking any sort of action, a way to tie it back to the business of the company. In the case of the Run for Something Better program, ING is one of the largest providers of retirement plans for teachers. Run for Something Better makes ING a visible part of the community and raises awareness of ING among the teacher community and boards of education.

Kelly concluded by noting that while ING can give a certain amount of money to the organizations involved in Run for Something Better, it is never enough, and the ING Foundation funds many other programs as well. In the interest of sustainability, ING recognized the need to get the public involved and, in 2006, created the Orange Laces program. For a $10 donation, donors receive a pair of orange shoe laces to demonstrate their support of this cause. Donors can visit the website (www.orangelaces.com) and designate the city that will receive their donation. In 2007, ING raised almost $400,000 in laces donations alone, and it is expected that this will increase in 2008 as awareness of the program expands.

OPEN DISCUSSION

In her presentation, Kelly noted the need for a "win-win" situation when a company decides to fund a program or establish a partnership. Expanding on this during the open discussion, White said that whether or not a particular program is funded is guided by the primary health conditions that WellPoint focuses on in support of the State Health Index. Courton Brown noted that companies are often inundated with proposals, and there needs to be a framework to assess and identify the proposals that are synergistic with the corporate organization. She said that many companies build their philanthropic strategies around their corporate expertise. Bank of America has an overarching set of philanthropic priorities, and a bank can choose to prioritize their funding for their own community. If health is an issue in one market, for example, that local branch can choose that as a priority. There is typically some sort of connection to the business of Bank of America with regard to what proposals are funded.

Another topic of discussion was the various compensation components that corporations provide to employees, specifically health benefits. Large companies often provide health benefits and are therefore a major contributor to addressing some of the socioeconomic determinants of health. A participant suggested that in many cases, however, lower-income employees do not receive such benefits, nor do employees of small companies, and that companies could do better at addressing disparities in health benefits. Brown said that benefits can exponentially add value to the compensation of the lowest paid employees. The ability to provide benefits is related to scale, and she questioned whether national organizations, or large regional organizations, would be able to bundle groups of employees to the point where the provision of some of these benefits could be offered.

7

Closing Comments

Before providing closing comments, Roundtable Chair Nicole Lurie opened the floor for discussion. Members of the Roundtable and of the workshop audience discussed sustainability of interventions, the link between spirituality and health, education of the next generation of physicians, and the need for a social movement to bring everyone together and address health disparities nationally.

OPEN DISCUSSION

Sustainability

Roundtable member America Bracho said that comprehensive interventions are needed in order to improve the health of our children. All of the elements discussed during the workshop converge to influence health outcomes. Including the community in the development of strategies brings not only common sense to the process, but also accountability. An engaged community will not allow a program to stop simply because the funding is gone, she said. One of the issues with developing comprehensive interventions is how the funding system works. Funding may be short term or categorical, or funders may only see value in new programs and may not continue to fund established programs. Bracho said that we need to work on place, bringing different designs to the communities, working with city engineers and health departments.

The models discussed during the workshop show how community involvement can lead to positive health outcomes, offered Roundtable member David Pryor, but he fears we will still be discussing the same issues about funding and sustainability 5 or 10 years from now. His recommendation was to have greater emphasis on developing an economic or political model that could produce sustainable change over a larger portion of the country, not just for isolated cities and isolated projects. We need to create a national platform so that, 10 years from now, we have moved beyond isolated successes to improvement in overall health indexes, Pryor noted.

Roundtable member James Krieger agreed, noting that we do not have the mechanisms to put programs in place beyond a boutique-type of approach, where there is a small amount of grant funding or a government program that may only last for 2 or 3 years. While communities may rise to the challenge to save a program, we cannot pass the responsibility to the communities who may also be victims of economic discrimination. We need to look for sustainable funding sources. About 90 percent of health related expenditures in this country are invested in the medical care sector, Krieger said, with the remainder going to support community-based projects and public health. In contrast, most of the determinants of disease, in particular determinants of health disparities, are not going to be addressed in the medical care sector but in the communities. Krieger suggested the Roundtable consider what could be done at the policy and financing levels to transfer resources from the medical health care sector to the public health and community sectors, so they have an ongoing sustainable resource base.

Another member of the Roundtable, Winston Wong, pointed out that no one addressed the myth of the "American Dream," that everyone has an equal chance for success in this country. There is a perception that if you are in despair in an economic or health sense, it is essentially your responsibility to pull yourself up by your bootstraps. Such countries as France, Sweden, and the United Kingdom have much more progressive understandings of the roles of communities, government, and organized groups with regard to accountability. Our programs are constructed based upon the flawed concept that Americans have some unique quality that enables us to be able to make personal progress toward this ideal of attaining wealth and fortune, or in this case, health.

Total Health: Spirituality and Education

Roundtable member Jennie Joe cited a recent research project involving the Native American community for whom spirituality is very important, and is not simply a religion, but something that provides a sense of cultural strength. It is a way of life and provides a sense of identity that is very important for the children. Many of us conducting research, she said, do not do justice to such cultural issues. Separation of church and state is ingrained in us, but the communities we work with are redefining spirituality in a very different context. Joe said she hopes for a future where the definition of who is healthy includes elements of spirituality.

One participant, who said she was a child care provider, agreed that the spiritual aspect of health deserves more attention. She also raised a concern about government takeover of child care, observing that before free programs were in place, children were well prepared when they entered kindergarten. But now, she believes that because of the poor quality of the free programs that are available, many children are entering special education kindergarten programs because they are not ready for school.

Roundtable member Alicia Dixon noted that another key factor that was not discussed in depth during the workshop was the importance of educating the health care workforce to be able to diminish or eliminate health disparities. We need to be training a different kind of physician. We can't keep training people in the same way, she said, and expect any kind of significant change in the systems that perpetuate the problems.

Creating a Health Movement

Workshop keynote speaker David Satcher expanded on the idea of creating a "movement." When enough people are moving in the same direction, he said, it draws the attention of policy makers. People involved in the movement, even though they may suffer, gain hope for change. Those engaged in a social movement change their own behavior and the behavior of others. He mentioned the WHO Commission on Social Determinants of Health, which is working to build a sustainable global movement to eliminate health inequities by targeting social determinants. He cited a program being undertaken in Chile to invest in early childhood education for the lowest 10 percent of the population in terms of socioeconomic level, providing day care and then education for children from 3 months of age onward. Such a program allows a parent to work, or a teenage mother to continue in school. The program also models good nutrition and fosters physical activity. How then, he asked, do we invest in a movement whereby we could really effect change in the United States? We need to develop a strategy to pull all of the people and groups engaged in this issue together, and to spread the message where it is most needed and where it will be most effective.

Roundtable member Mildred Thompson concurred with Satcher regarding the need for a movement, and suggested that in order to create a movement there needs to be a common vision about how this is a problem for all of us, and that solving it benefits all of us. The issue needs to be carefully framed and communicated, using language that does not create a perception of "us and them." As long as we see health disparities as being "their" problem, people are not going to see themselves as being part of the solution.

Workshop attendee Marian Dennis followed up by noting that health disparities are the result of socioeconomic determinants of health, driven in large part by poverty. With regard to framing the issue, disparities in health are not limited to ethnic and racial minorities, but also affect a significant number of people in the United States who face poverty. She suggested that there is a currently a window of opportunity to start a movement because many people who didn't think of themselves as vulnerable are now becoming more vulnerable. Many people who have viewed themselves as middle class are worried about losing their jobs and homes.

The struggles facing immigrants were raised by another participant, who said they want the best for their families but often cannot afford health care or insurance, or education beyond public school.

CONCLUSION

In closing, Lurie noted that the impending recession has the potential to make disparities much greater. With the many current discussions about race and gender and politics, Lurie said that disparities in health are not about Republicans and Democrats, or men and women. It is, in part, a generational issue. It is about what our country and the world are going to be like for our children. That is really the theme of the workshop, she said. The way we invest in our children has incredible implications for the health of our country, the well-being of our citizens, the productivity of our country, global competitiveness, and America's place in the world. What happens in the womb, and in the early years of life, have a great impact on lifelong health. Lurie noted that it behooves all of us to bring these issues into the public discourse. She cited the PBS video series presented by Thompson as an important step in this direction. Lurie urged participants to be active in their own communities, including bringing up these issues with local candidates, regardless what level of office they are running for. Challenge people to think about creative solutions, she said. Let people know that there is a movement coming and that they need to get on board.

A

Workshop Agenda

Investing in Children's Health:
A Community Approach to Addressing Health Disparities

Roundtable on Health Disparities
Public Meeting
Morehouse School of Medicine's
Louis W. Sullivan National Center for Primary Care Auditorium

720 Westview Drive, S.W.
Atlanta, Georgia
January 24, 2008

8:30 a.m—Welcome
Dr. John E. Maupin Jr., President
Morehouse School of Medicine

Dr. Gary Nelson, President
Healthcare Georgia Foundation
Member, Roundtable on Health Disparities

8:40 a.m.—Keynote Address
Dr. David Satcher, 16th Surgeon General of the United States,
Director of the Satcher Health Leadership Institute at Morehouse
School of Medicine

9:00 a.m.—Investments to Promote Children's Health: A Systematic
Literature Review and Economic Analysis of Interventions in the
Preschool Period
Dr. Bernard Guyer, Professor
Johns Hopkins Bloomberg School of Public Health
Clinical Practice and Community Building: Addressing Racial
Disparities in Healthy Child Development
Dr. Charles Bruner, Executive Director
Child Family Policy Center

10:00 a.m.—Break

10:15 a.m.—From Policy to Practice: How Policy Changes Can Affect Children's Lives
> Christine Ferguson, Associate Research Professor of Health Policy
> The George Washington University
> Yvonne Sanders-Butler, Principal
> Browns Mill Elementary and Magnet for High Achievers

11:15 a.m.—Audience Discussion

11:45 a.m.—Lunch—Auditorium Lobby

1:00 p.m.—Unnatural Causes: Is Inequality Making Us Sick?
> Mildred Thompson, Senior Director
> PolicyLink

1:45 p.m.—Community Development Approaches: Overcoming Challenges, Striving for Change
> Veda Johnson
> Whitefoord Community Program, and Assistant Professor in the Department of Pediatrics, Emory University School of Medicine
>
> Marshall Kreuter, Professor of Public Health
> Georgia State University
>
> Wayne Giles, Director
> Division of Adult and Community Health
> Center for Disease Control and Prevention

3:00 p.m.—Break

3:15 p.m.—Do Businesses Have a Role in Improving Communities or Improving Children's Lives?
> Sandra White, Medical Director
> WellPoint, Inc.
>
> Maureen Kelly, Director of Community Relations and Vice President
> ING Foundation

Michele Courton Brown, Senior Vice President of Charitable Management Services, Bank of America

4:15 p.m.—Audience Discussion

5:00 p.m.—Adjourn

B

Biosketches of Presenters and Authors

Michelle Courton Brown is Senior Vice President and National Practice Director for Bank of America's Philanthropic Management Group. In that capacity, she provides expert philanthropic advice to high net-worth clients, and strategic guidance for the business group's professional development, sales support, and thought leadership initiatives. Formerly, Ms. Courton Brown served as a Market Director for Philanthropic Management, leading a team of professionals who served the client service, fiduciary, administrative, and philanthropic advisory needs of high net-worth individuals, families, foundations and nonprofit institutions.

From 1999 to 2002, Ms. Courton Brown served as founding President of the FleetBoston Financial Foundation, which contributed over $25 million annually to charitable endeavors. Previously, she served as Director of Corporate Contributions for BankBoston and Executive Director of the Travelers Insurance Companies Foundation. In 2004, Michele coauthored "Just Money: A Critique of Contemporary American Philanthropy."

A graduate of Boston University, Ms. Courton Brown is a civic leader, serving on the boards of numerous local and national nonprofit boards including serving as the chair of Roxbury Community College, the chair of the Chestnut Hill School, and as a trustee of Faulkner Hospital, Boys and Girls Clubs of Boston, and YouthBuild USA.

Charles Bruner, M.A., Ph.D., serves as Executive Director of the Child and Family Policy Center, a nonprofit organization established in 1989 "to better link research and policy on issues vital to children and families." He holds an M.A. and Ph.D. in political science from Stanford University, and received his B.A. from Macalester College. Dr. Bruner served 12 years as a state legislator in Iowa.

Through the Child and Family Policy Center, Bruner provides technical assistance to states, communities, and foundations on child and family issues. Dr. Bruner's current interests relate to developing more neighborhood-based service systems that integrate professional and voluntary supports and serve in community-building as well as family-strengthening roles. The Child and Family Policy Center also leads the Des Moines Making Connections activities in the area of Children Healthy and Prepared for Success in School (CHAPSS).

Yvonne Sanders-Butler, Ed.D., is the President and Founder of Ennovy, Inc., a company that provides comprehensive health and wellness intervention, consultation, and support. She is a nutritional advocate, consultant, and motivational speaker promoting healthy living for life. Dr. Sanders-Butler is also the author of *Naturally Yours and More Gourmet Desserts, Dessert Lovers' Choice,* and the soon to be released *Healthy Kids, Smart Kids.*

Dr. Sanders-Butler serves as the principal of Browns Mill Elementary and Magnet School for High Achievers, the only elementary school in DeKalb County named a Georgia 2005 School of Excellence and a National Blue Ribbon School. Since 1999, it has been the only sugar-free school in the state of Georgia.

Dr. Sanders-Butler has appeared on ABC News, Fox News, CNN News, the Martha Stewart Show, local and national radio stations, and in various national, regional and city publications such as *Essence, Southern Living Magazine, Upscale, Women Health Fitness, Sister to Sister, Black Enterprise,* the *Atlanta Journal Constitution* newspaper, *Tom Joyner, BAW News,* and other media outlets to discuss and promote healthy living for life. She also conducted a 3-month wellness behavior management program at Jackson State University in Jackson, Mississippi, to improve student health and well-being. Dr. Sanders-Butler received her B.S. degree in mass communications from Jackson State University, her masters degree in counseling from State University of West Georgia, a specialist degree in administration from Jackson State University, and her doctorate in educational leadership from Sarasota University.

Christine Ferguson, J.D., is an associate research professor at the George Washington University School of Public Health and Health Services' Department of Health Policy. From 1981 to 1995, Ferguson served as counsel and deputy chief of staff to the late U.S. Senator John H. Chafee (R-RI), where she led his wide-ranging efforts to reform national health and social policy for all Americans, with a special focus on health services to medically underserved populations. Ferguson served as secretary of the Rhode Island

Department of Human Services from 1995 to 2001. In this capacity, she oversaw nearly one-third of the state's annual budget. As commissioner of the Massachusetts Department of Public Health under Governor Mitt Romney from 2003 to 2005, Ferguson led the administration's efforts in the areas of emergency preparedness, substance abuse services, medical errors reduction, and early childhood education and child care. Most recently, Ferguson served as president of First Focus, a special initiative funded by the David and Lucile Packard Foundation and the Atlantic Philanthropies. A graduate of the University of Michigan and the Washington College of Law at American University, Ferguson currently serves as a member of the Board on Children, Youth, and Families of the National Academy of Sciences and has served in a leadership capacity at the National Academy for State Health Policy and other organizations.

Wayne Giles, M.D., joined the Centers for Disease Control and Prevention (CDC) in July 1992. He is currently the director of the Division of Adult and Community Health at the National Center for Chronic Disease Prevention and Health Promotion. He holds a bachelors degree in biology from Washington University, a masters in epidemiology from the University of Maryland, and an M.D. from Washington University. He has completed residencies in both internal medicine (University of Alabama at Birmingham) and preventive medicine (University of Maryland).

Dr. Giles' past work experience has included studies examining the prevalence of hypertension in Africa, clinical trials evaluating the effectiveness of cholesterol-lowering agents, and studies examining racial differences in the incidence of stroke. Dr. Giles currently directs programmatic and research activities in arthritis, aging, health care utilization, and racial and ethnic disparities in health within the Division of Adult and Community Health at CDC.

Dr. Giles has authored more than 100 articles in peer-reviewed journals and has authored several book chapters. He has been the recipient of numerous awards, including the Distinguished Researcher Award by the International Society on Hypertension in Blacks and the Jeffrey P. Koplan Award by CDC.

Bernard Guyer, M.D., M.P.H., is Zanvyl Krieger Professor of Children's Health, in the Department of Population, Family, and Reproductive Health at the Johns Hopkins Bloomberg School of Public Health. Guyer trained in pediatrics and preventive medicine and served as an E.I.S. officer at the CDC. From 1979 to 1986, Dr. Guyer directed the Maternal and Child Health (MCH) agency in the Massachusetts Department of Public Health.

Dr. Guyer has been active in maternal and child health policy at the national, state, and local levels. He is a member of the Institute of Medicine and chairs the Board on Children, Youth, and Families at the Institute of Medicine. Guyer chaired the Maryland Commission on Infant Mortality, served on the board of the Baltimore Healthy Start Program, and participates in the Baltimore Better Babies Leadership in Action Program (BLAP). He is a member of the U.S. Department of Health and Human Services Secretary's Advisory Committee on Infant Mortality.

Dr. Guyer's areas of research include low birth weight and infant mortality, child development and pediatric care, childhood injury and injury prevention, and urban health. He was principal investigator of the National Evaluation of the Healthy Steps for Young Children program. He has directed several needs assessments, including those for the Massachusetts Title V/MCH Block Grant and the Baltimore City Healthy Start Program. He served as Senior Academic Advisor to the Johns Hopkins University Urban Health Institute and is the author of more than 200 published papers. Dr. Guyer received the "Golden Apple" Teaching Award in 2003 from the school's students, as well as the 2003 Martha May Eliot Award from the American Public Health Association.

Veda Charmaine Johnson, M.D., is the Director of Community- and School-Based Clinics for the Department of Pediatrics at Emory University School of Medicine in Atlanta, Georgia. She also serves as Medical Director of the Whitefoord Elementary and Sammye E. Coan Middle School Health Clinics and the Lindbergh Women and Children's Health Clinic. She received a bachelor of science degree from Alma College and completed her first 2 years of medical school at the School of Medicine at Morehouse College. She received her medical degree from Emory University School, where she also completed a residency in pediatrics. After completing an additional year as Chief Resident, Dr. Johnson served a 4-year obligation with the National Health Service Corp in Meridian, Mississippi, where she served as Medical Director at the Meridian Community Health Center.

In 1992, Dr. Johnson accepted a position at Emory University to develop a comprehensive school-based clinic in the Atlanta school system. After receiving funding from the Department of Health and Human Services' Healthy Schools, Healthy Communities (HSHC) program, the school clinic opened its doors in November 1994. Additional federal funding was secured to expand school-based health services into the community's Coan Middle School. This clinic became operational in the fall of 1999.

In addition to serving as Medical Director and Program Director for the Whitefoord and Coan School Clinics, she is an assistant professor of pediatrics at Emory University School of Medicine and acts as the Medical Director for community-based pediatric primary care clinics affiliated with the Grady Health System. Dr. Johnson serves on the boards of the National

Association of School-Based Health Centers and the Good Samaritan Health Center, a health center catering to the poor and homeless of Atlanta.

Marshall Kreuter, Ph.D., M.P.H. (Hon.), is a Professor in the Public Health Institute at Georgia State University in Atlanta. His primary interests are in the areas of strategic planning, implementation, evaluation of community-based public health programs, and the assessment of the relationship between social capital and community-based health improvement initiatives. In 2000, Dr. Kreuter retired as a Distinguished Scientist/Fellow at CDC in Atlanta, where he served in several key leadership roles: Director of the Division of Health Education, the first director of the Division of Chronic Disease Control and Community Intervention, and Director of the Prevention Research Centers program. While at CDC, Dr. Kreuter and colleagues refined the epidemiologic study of physical activity, initiated research and programs focused on the early detection of breast cancer, developed a stronger emphasis on school health, and created the Planned Approach to Community Health program. Dr. Kreuter received a Ph.D. from the University of Utah, completed a postdoctoral fellowship at the Johns Hopkins School of Hygiene and Public Health, and was awarded an honorary master of public health degree from the University of Las Palmas de Gran Canaria in Spain. He has authored several books and papers on health promotion and is the recipient of numerous awards, among them the John P. McGovern Medal for distinguished contributions to health education and the Distinguished Fellow Award, the highest honor awarded by the Society for Public Health Education.

Edward Schor, M.D., is Vice President of the Child Development and Preventive Care program at the Commonwealth Fund. Dr. Schor, a pediatrician, has held a number of positions in pediatric practice, academic pediatrics, health services research, and public health. Immediately prior to joining the fund in 2002, he served as medical director for the Iowa Department of Public Health, Division of Family and Community Health. Earlier in his career, Dr. Schor was medical director of the Chesapeake Health Plan in Baltimore, Maryland, Director of the Division of General Pediatrics at the University of New Mexico, Program Director for Medical Education and Improving Functional Outcomes and Well-Being with the Henry J. Kaiser Family Foundation, and Director of the Functional Outcomes Program at the New England Medical Center. He received postdoctoral training in social and behavioral sciences and has a special interest in the social determinants of child health and family functioning.

Dr. Schor is editor of the book, *Caring for Your School-Age Child*, and has chaired both the Committee on Early Childhood, Adoption, and Dependent care and the national Task Force on the Family for the American Academy of Pediatrics. He also has served on the Maternal and Child Health Bureau's Child Health Survey Technical Panel, consulted for the National Center for Infancy and Early Childhood Health Policy, and co-chaired the IHCI/National Initiative for Children's Healthcare Quality on the topic of improving health care for children in foster care. He received the 2006 John C. MacQueen Award from the Association of Maternal and Child Health Programs. Dr. Schor has been a member of the faculties of several major university medical schools and schools of public health. He has also served on the editorial boards of a number of pediatric journals.

Sandra White, M.D., M.B.A., is the Medical Director of Medical Management with Blue Cross/Blue Shield of Georgia and is responsible for case management, utilization management, and quality initiatives related to health disparities, breast cancer, and specialty pharmacy. She participates with network management and provider relations for assigned hospitals and geographic areas. Dr. White's areas of interest include health and disease management and improving consumer understanding of health-related information to improve health literacy, and facilitate self-management. Dr. White received her B.S. degree from City College of City University of New York, her M.D. degree from Mount Sinai School of Medicine, and her M.B.A. from Kennesaw State University. She is a diplomate of the American Board of Internal Medicine and Rheumatology, and a diplomate of the American Board of Quality Assurance and Utilization Review Physicians with Certifications in Managed Care.

C

Resources

The following list is provided for those interested in learning more about the model programs and other resources mentioned throughout the workshop. The IOM Roundtable on Health Disparities does not endorse any particular programs, publications, or websites.

MODEL PROGRAMS

Accountable Communities: Healthy Together (ACHT)
http://publichealth.gsu.edu/accountable.asp

The Dirty Truth Campaign (an initiative of ACHT)
http://www.dirtytruth.org/index.html

Healthy Kids, Smart Kids
http://www.healthykidssmartkids.com/

Help Me Grow (Connecticut)
http://www.ct.gov/CTF/cwp/view.asp?a=1786&q=296676

ING Run for Something Better
http://orangelaces.com

Racial and Ethnic Approaches to Community Health (REACH)
http://www.cdc.gov/reach

RIte Care (Rhode Island Medicare Manage Care program)
http://www.ritecare.ri.gov/

WellPoint, Inc.
http://www.wellpoint.com

Whitefoord Community Program
http://www.whitefoord.org/

FUNDING

Corporate

Bank of America, Corporate Philanthropy
http://www.bankofamerica.com/foundation

ING Foundation Grants
http://www.ing-usa.com/us/aboutING/CorporateCitizenship/
INGFoundationGrants/index.htm

Government

Health Resources and Services Administration
http://www.hrsa.gov

National Center on Minority Health and Health Disparities
http://ncmhd.nih.gov

State Children's Health Insurance Program
http://www.cms.hhs.gov/home/schip.asp

ADDITIONAL RESOURCES

Healthy People 2010
http://www.healthypeople.gov

Photovoice
http://www.photovoice.org

Unnatural Causes (PBS documentary)
http://www.unnaturalcauses.org

D

Special Presentation: Unnatural Causes

In addition to the presentations and panel discussions described in the report, Mildred Thompson of PolicyLink, co-chair of the Roundtable, provided the workshop participants with an opportunity to preview a segment of a forthcoming PBS documentary series entitled "Unnatural Causes: Is Inequality Making Us Sick?," which explores socioeconomic and racial inequities in health. The purpose of the preview was to educate Roundtable members and the audience about the root of causes of health disparities but more importantly to foster discussion about how the documentary can be used as a tool to stimulate action in communities and organizations. The first segment in the series aired on March 27, 2008, on PBS stations.[1]

The segment screened at the workshop, entitled "When the Bough Breaks," addressed the disproportionate infant mortality rates of babies born to African American women. One striking conclusion from this segment that Thompson highlighted was that African American women with college degrees have worse birth outcomes than non-Hispanic white women who are high school dropouts (mortality rates of 10.2 per 1,000 versus 9.9 per 1,000, respectively). Thompson also drew attention to the role of stress in poor health outcomes, citing the example of the married African American lawyer that was featured in the segment shown. The video dis-

---

[1] The documentary and associated toolkit, produced by California Newsreel in association with Vital Pictures, and presented by the National Minority Consortia of public television, can be found at http://www.unnaturalcauses.org.

cussed the stress and racism that may have contributed to the premature birth of her infant.

After viewing the segment, a member of the audience commented that while the segment focused on African American women, similar outcomes are observed with Hispanic women, most dramatically among Puerto Rican women, and opined that this affects all women of color. Disparities within ethnic groups were also discussed, as some subgroups within Latino and Asian ethnic groups suffer from higher rates of illness and disease than other subgroups within the same ethnic group. For example, recent Mexican immigrants, despite being poorer, have better health than other Latinos already living in the United States.

Another participant commented that while direct implications of racism in health care are easy to see, there are also indirect effects of institutional racism, specifically neglect. She highlighted the increasing prevalence of HIV among African Americans and Latinos and the associated lack of money for programs to address HIV in these populations as an example of such neglect.

One example of a successful community initiative in Flint, Michigan, part of the REACH program, was cited by another participant. Workshops conducted in the community bring people together to discuss what is needed in terms of undoing racism. They are having productive conversations, and change is occurring, the participant noted. For example, over the last 6 years, a 25 percent reduction in infant mortality among African American women has been observed. Another participant noted, however, that it is only the REACH program in Flint that has seen such a reduction in infant mortality.

Although overall infant mortality rates have decreased over the years, they are still disproportionately high among African American and other women of color. Thompson urged participants to continue the dialogue in their communities and organizations to address disparities especially across races, sectors, and genders.

E

Clinical Health Care Practice and Community Building: Addressing Racial Disparities in Healthy Child Development

Charles H. Bruner, Ph.D., and Edward L. Schor, M.D.

INTRODUCTION AND SYNOPSIS

Pronounced disparities exist by race and ethnicity in child and adolescent health across a range of health conditions and access to health services. Addressing these child health disparities is particularly important, as childhood and adolescence establish health trajectories that extend throughout a person's life span.[1]

These disparities in child health conditions by race and ethnicity also co-occur with other disparities in child outcomes—from educational achievement to child welfare and justice system involvement. This high degree of co-occurrence warrants attention to identifying some common etiology for these disparities.[2]

Clearly, good child health involves

- timely and appropriate (and therefore culturally sensitive) medical care for illness and injury, and screening to detect and treat congenital abnormalities and chronic as well as acute health conditions;
- good hygiene, nutrition, and exercise;
- stable and nurturing families who provide constant and consistent supervision;
- safe environments that do not contain toxic elements;[3]
- social institutions that reinforce healthy lifestyles and behaviors and provide opportunities for growth and development; and
- social and psychological supports that foster resiliency and positive identity.[4]

Healthy child development that results in educational and social success similarly involves the same set of points, particularly when social institutions are defined to include schools and their educational components. These points provide the basis for that common etiology to achieving both good child health and healthy child development.

In the United States, the first two points on this list generally are considered to be subject to influence by the health care system through the primary pediatric practitioner. The last four points generally are considered to be primarily influenced by the child's family and community and their network of supports, with some role from public health on environmental health conditions, a role for schools for educational development, and a role for law enforcement for public safety.[5]

This paper argues that such distinctions and segmentations of responsibility can miss opportunities for addressing child health disparities by race and ethnicity. In fact, child health practitioners[6] and their institutions can play a contributing role in supporting child health and healthy child development across all these points. As an example, Figure 3-2 shows that when the pediatric practitioner's role is broadly defined and practiced, the set of healthy child development outcomes that should be at least partially addressed through well-child care for young children involves identifying potential concerns on all these points and at least beginning to address them.[7]

Defining child health and the responsibilities of the health care community broadly is particularly important in distressed or vulnerable neighborhoods, where child health outcomes are poorest and where children of color disproportionately live.[8] While there is a limited clinical research base regarding the effectiveness of more holistic pediatric approaches to healthy child development, there is also little within current research to indicate an inability to develop such pediatric practice.[9] Further, there are promising programs with evidence of success in improving health outcomes and reducing disparities that deserve attention and support, particularly as they connect children and families to other community-building activities. Two such programs—Help Me Grow in Connecticut and the Eastside Partnership for Families in Richmond, Virginia—are described as examples of exemplary efforts to combine clinical practices with community-building ones. Linking clinical practice with community-building efforts offers promise in both improving child health and children's healthy development, but requires explicit attention to the role that child health practitioners should play in supporting other organizations in leading community-building efforts. Expanding the knowledge and practice base on effective strategies that combine clinical and community-building strategies also requires evaluation approaches that extend beyond traditional clinical trials as ways to attribute causality and measure impact.

DISPARITIES IN HEALTHY CHILD DEVELOPMENT
BY RACE AND ETHNICITY

There is a large, although fragmented, array of data that shows profound disparities in child health outcomes, as well as access to health services, by race and ethnicity. These disparities start even before birth and extend through adolescence and into adulthood. That disparities differ among different racial and ethnic groups depending upon the child outcome is also an important point in understanding the origins and determinants of disparity. Figure 3-1 provides prevalence data on several child and adolescent health measures, broken out for the three largest racial and ethnic groupings in America—white non-Hispanic, African American, and Hispanic (see Table E-1 for a more extensive list of child health and other outcomes by these population groups). Disparities also exist for Native American children and, on some measures, for Asian and Pacific Islander children, but these are not shown in this figure. Figure 3-1 further provides prevalence data on measures of educational and social development and on family factors and characteristics.

As Figure 3-1 indicates, there are consistent and marked disparities in child health outcomes and access to child health services, with African American children faring far worse than white, non-Hispanic children on almost every measure. With the exception of birth outcomes and child and adolescent mortality, Hispanic children also fare much worse on most measures than white, non-Hispanic children.[10] As has been frequently noted, the African American infant mortality rate is equivalent to the rates in many developing countries. Most other child health indicators among African American and Hispanic children show similar degrees of disparity when compared with White, non-Hispanic children.

Table E-1 shows that these child health disparities are similar in size to those found for educational and social outcomes. In other words, disparities related to healthy child development and school success are equally profound to those related to specific health conditions. Finally, the family and community factors for African American and Hispanic children are very different from those for white, non-Hispanic children. In respect to wealth (and therefore the ability to invest in one's future) and geographic location, the differences are even more pronounced across race and ethnicity than for most of the health and healthy development outcomes experienced by children. In 2000, for instance, median household net worth for white non-Hispanic households was $79,400, compared with $7,500 for African American and $9,750 for Hispanic households—a 10-fold difference, much greater than when annual income is compared. (See Table E-1 for more information.)[11]

Overall, this collection of data points to the importance of looking

TABLE E-1 Child Health Disparities in Context: Selected Indicators of Child Health, Healthy Development, and Family and Community

Child Health Indicators	White NH	Black NH	Hispanic	Source
Infant mortality (1,000 live births)	5.7	13.8	5.6	A
Low birth weight	7.2%	13.4%	6.8%	A
Elevated blood-lead levels	2.6%	4.3%	3.1%	B
Current asthma prevalence (under 18)	8.0%	13.0%	8.6%	C
New AIDS cases 13–17/100,000	.1	4.0	.5	D
Child (1–14) death rate/100,000	19	29	18	A
Teen death (15–19) rate/100,000	63	81	64	A
6–11 Overweight	11.8%	19.5%	23.7%	E
19–29 Overweight	12.7%	23.6%	23.4%	E
Child health indicators				
No health insurance coverage 0–17	6.4%	6.9%	19.5%	D
No reported specific source of care 0–17	3.3%	5.8%	24.1%	D
Late/no entry into prenatal care	11.0%	24.1%	23.5%	D
No dental visit (2–17)	41.4%	63.2%	63.3%	D
Immunizations not complete (19–35 mo)	16.7%	25.5%	21.3%	D
Asthma hospital admissions (0–4)/100,000	15.3	120.0	54.0	D
Hospital admin ped. gastrointes. (0–17)/100,000	81.7	84.1	108.9	D
Healthy Child Development Indicators/Education				
Below basic 4th-grade reading proficiency	22%	54%	50%	F
Below basic 8th-grade math proficiency	18%	53%	45%	F
15–24 dropout rates	6.0%	10.4%	22.4%	G
Noncompletion of high school	24.1%	48.8%	46.8%	H

Healthy Child Development—Other

Youth (16–19) not in school or working	6%	12%	A
Foster care placement (0–17)/1,000	4.9	6.5	I
Males (20–24) in state/federal prison/1,000	9.5	24.9	J

Family and Community Indicators

Children in poverty	11%	29%	A
No parent employed year-round	27%	39%	A
Children in single-parent families	23%	36%	A
Teen (15–19) birth rate/1,000 females	2.6%	8.3%	A
Living in high-risk neighborhood	1.7%	25.3%	K
Median household net worth	$74,900	$9,750	L

Child Population

2000 population	44,027,087	12,342,259
Percentage of total child population	60.9%	17.1%
Projected 2020 population	42,459,109	18,923,344
Percentage of total	52.9%	23.6%

SOURCES:

A. Annie E. Casey Foundation. 2007. *2007 kids count data book: State profiles of child well-being.* Baltimore, MD: Annie E. Casey Foundation.

B. Centers for Disease Control. 2005. Blood lead levels—United States, 1999-2002. *Morbidity and Mortality Weekly Report* 54(20):513-516. http://www.cdc.gov/mmwr/preview/ mmwrhtml/mm5420a.htm.

C. Centers for Disease Control. 2006. *National Health Interview Survey data—2005 data.* Table 4-1. http://www.cdc.gov/asthma/nhis/default. htm.

TABLE E-1 Continued

D. Agency for Healthcare Research and Quality. 2006. *National Health Care Disparities Report.* Appendix D: Data Tables. http://www.ahrq.gov/qual/nhdr06/index.html#MCH.

E. Weight Awareness. 2007. *Ethnicities and childhood overweight and obesity problems.* http:/www.weightawareness.com/topics/doc.xml?doc_id=1179&am.

F. National Center for Education Statistics. 2007. *National Assessment of Educational Progress scores—2007.* http://nationsreportcard.gov.

G. National Center for Education Statistics. 2005. *Status dropout rates for 15–24 year-olds,* October 2005. http://nces.ed.gov/pubs2007/dropout05.

H. Urban Institute. 2004. *Who graduates: Who doesn't.* http://www.urban.org/Uploaded PDF/410934_ WhoGraduates.pdf.

I. Adoption and Foster Care Analysis and Reporting System. 2004–2005. *Prevalence data by race.* http://www.acf.gov/programs/cb/stats_research/afcars/tar/report13.htm. This prevalence data was divided by census data on the number of children of different ethnicities to come up with percentages.

J. Bureau of Justice Statistics. 2005. *Prisoners in 2005.* http://oip.usdoj.gov/bjs/pub/pdf/p05.pdf.

K. Bruner, C., M. Wright, and S. Tirmizi. 2007. *Village building and school readiness: Closing opportunity gaps in a diverse society.* Des Moines, IA: State Early Childhood Policy Technical Assistance Network.

L. Orzechowski, S., and P. Sepielli. 2003. *Net worth and asset ownership of households: 1998 and 2000. Current population reports.* Washington, DC: U.S. Census. Pp. 70-88.

for underlying causal underpinnings for disparities that, for child health outcomes, extends beyond health insurance coverage and clinical care. The size of the disparities on health and healthy development measures cannot be attributed to health coverage alone. This involves exploring family, social institution, and community factors. The specific issue of geography, or place, is discussed in the next section of this paper.

PLACE AS AN IMPORTANT ELEMENT IN CHILD HEALTH DISPARITIES

The bank robber Willie Sutton is quoted as saying that he robbed banks because that was where the money was. Similarly, improving child health and reducing health disparities by race and ethnicity involve strategies that are delivered at the community level, where families can go to local facilities for their children's health needs. When children are very young, family time spent together and associations are much more likely to be geographically bound to a physical neighborhood. Research findings on neighborhood effects on child and family outcomes independent of individual child and family characteristics are mixed.[12] However, it is clear that place matters in developing strategies to reduce health disparities, if only because children of color, and particularly children of color with other economic and social factors that can contribute to poor health outcomes, disproportionately reside in certain neighborhoods and communities.

This is very clear from an analysis of 2000 census data of all 65,000 census tracts in the United States on 10 factors associated with their "child-raising vulnerability."[13] The 10 factors available from the census data were selected to provide indicators related to education, social structure, employment, and wealth. Each tract was categorized according to the number of factors upon which its data showed a high degree of vulnerability (one standard deviation or more from the mean). Figure 3-3 provides information that shows differences across census tracts with the presence of different numbers of vulnerability factors.

As Figure 3-3 shows, with the exception of wage income, the difference between census tracts with no risk factors and those with six or more risk factors are profound, with rates from two-and-one-quarter to nine times greater in the high-vulnerability tracts. The experience of children growing up in these high-vulnerability tracts is almost certainly very different than the experience of children growing up in those with little or no vulnerability. Except for the South, these high-vulnerability tracts are concentrated in metropolitan, largely inner-city, neighborhoods, with the highest concentrations of these in the Northeast.

While pointing to the importance of place-based approaches to improving child health and healthy child development, particularly important for this report is the fact that these high vulnerability census tracts also are very disproportionately populated by persons of color. Table E-2 shows the racial and ethnic composition for census tracts with different numbers of vulnerability factors.

As Table E-2 indicates, while 83.2 percent of the persons residing in tracts with no vulnerability factors are white, non-Hispanic, only 17.6 percent of the persons residing in tracts with six or more vulnerability factors are white, non-Hispanic. As a percentage of their overall population in the United States, only 1.7 percent of white, non-Hispanics in the country live in the highest vulnerability census tracts (six or more vulnerability factors), while 20.3 percent of blacks and 25.3 percent of Hispanics live in those tracts. Only 7.7 percent of white, non-Hispanics live in census tracts with three or more vulnerability factors, while 46.4 percent of blacks and 50.3 percent of Hispanics live in those neighborhoods.

In short, successful efforts to reduce child health and other disparities by race and ethnicity will have to make substantial gains within these high-vulnerability census tracts, simply due to the very substantial percentage of the child population of color that resides in those tracts.

In addition, however, available evidence also shows that the health and healthy development child outcomes are the poorest for both African American and Hispanic children who live within these census tracts.[14] Developing successful efforts in these tracts and neighborhoods likely requires considerable attention to addressing environmental and neighborhood,[15] as well as individual and family, conditions that exist there, which also have been referred to as "toxic stress" that harms brain development in children.[16] Neighborhood conditions include physical indicators such as levels of safety and exposure to environmental toxins, but also role models and social ties and connections that look out for children. Individual and family conditions include economic and educational conditions, but also levels of stress and child nurturing patterns. Conceptually, these factors interact as well, as neighborhood conditions contribute to or mitigate against family stress and provide or fail to provide nurturing activities and modeling for parents.

TOWARD A THEORY OF CHANGE IN ADDRESSING CHILD HEALTH DISPARITIES

The size and consistency of the disparities shown in Figure 3-1 suggest that there are at least some common underlying elements that contribute to and will need to be addressed in order to reduce or eliminate child health and healthy development disparities. The information in Table E-2 and Figure 3-3 suggests that neighborhood-based, as well as individual-based, strategies may need to be developed to address these disparities, at least in high-child vulnerability neighborhoods.

TABLE E-2 Racial Composition of Census Tracts by Child-Raising Vulnerability Status

Racial Composition	All Census Tracts	No Vulnerability Factors	1–2 Vulnerability Factors	3–5 Vulnerability Factors	6–10 Vulnerability Factors
% White non-Hispanic	69.8	83.2	67.0	37.4	17.6
% Black	12.5	6.2	13.4	28.2	38.0
% Asian	4.1	3.7	5.1	4.4	3.4
% Hispanic	12.5	6.1	13.3	28.1	39.4
% Am. Indian/Native Alaskan	0.8	0.5	0.9	1.4	1.2
% Native Hawaiian and other PI	0.2	0.2	0.2	0.2	0.2
% Other	0.2	0.1	0.2	0.2	0.2
Total	100	100	100	100	100
Proportion of race in tract					
% White non-Hispanic	100	69.6	22.7	6.0	1.7
% Black	100	29.1	25.2	25.4	20.3
% Asian	100	52.6	29.7	12.3	5.5
% Hispanic	100	28.6	25.0	25.0	25.3
% Am. Indian/Native Alaskan	100	40.3	27.6	21.0	11.1
% Native Hawaiian and other PI	100	50.6	29.9	13.4	6.1
% Other	100	47.6	26.6	15.4	10.4

SOURCE: Census data, 2000.

Increasingly, initiatives designed to produce community-level changes in child and family outcomes have adopted a "theory of change" approach to evaluation.[17] The purpose of applying a theory of change is to identify assumptions that underlie the belief that the strategies developed will lead to producing community-level changes in the desired child and family outcomes. An evaluation design can then be developed to test the different assumptions upon which the strategies are based.

As stated in the introduction, good child health and healthy child development involves

- timely and appropriate (and therefore culturally sensitive) medical care for illness and injury and screening to detect and treat congenital abnormalities and chronic as well as acute health conditions;
- good hygiene, nutrition, and exercise;
- stable and nurturing families who provide constant and consistent supervision;
- safe environments that do not contain toxic elements;
- social institutions that reinforce healthy lifestyles and behaviors and provide opportunities for growth and development; and
- social and psychological supports that foster resiliency and positive identity.

These points can form the basis for a theory of change, as everything on this list is malleable to some degree.[18] Clearly, most children receive most of what they need most of the time to produce good, if not optimal, health and healthy development outcomes. The issue is to identify where children are not receiving what they need and then develop strategies to ensure they receive it. Box E-1 provides the assumptions for such a theory of change to address these disparities.

Clearly, there is a research as well as a theoretical (and common sense) base for each of the assumptions in this theory of change. There is substantial research on assumptions one and two that show there are a set of interrelated underlying factors beyond the child's own constitution and genetic make-up that contribute to good child health and healthy development. These extend from clinical research on the impact of medical interventions, to anthropological and sociological research on the role of the family in child development, to resiliency and risk and protective factor research on the importance of social institutions and social and psychological supports to healthy development.[19] Further, all these factors are malleable to some extent.

There also is substantial evidence that while child health insurance coverage and the provision of clinical pediatric services play a role in improving child health and reducing health disparities, social and environmental fac-

---

BOX E-1
Theory of Change Set of Testable Assumptions for Strengthening Pediatric Practices to Reduce Disparities in Healthy Child Development

1. Pronounced, but malleable, disparities in child health exist by race/ethnicity, which correspond with similar pronounced disparities in educational achievement, justice system involvement, and income and wealth.
2. These disparities are not separate and distinct, but are interconnected, requiring strategies for addressing them that need to recognize and address some of their common underlying causes.
3. Because it is almost universally used by young children, child health care practice offers an important entry point that can be used to identify and begin to address these underlying causes.
4. This requires a more holistic and culturally congruent approach to primary, preventive, and developmental pediatric care than is currently in practice from a clinical perspective, coupled with effective referrals to other services and supports at the community level that contribute to community building.
5. Developing such strategies is particularly important in distressed neighborhoods, where children of color disproportionately reside and where environmental factors most threaten child health and development, with actions taken to increase the social capital and reduce the environmental risk within those neighborhoods.
6. The result of developing such strategies will be to significantly improve both specific measures of child health and to improve broader measures of healthy child development.

---

tors weigh much more heavily in producing current disparities.[20] Further, although often not considered as an objective or goal (i.e., the dependent variable in a regression equation), there is at least case study evidence that child health insurance coverage and clinical pediatric services can play a role in improving healthy child development and educational and social outcomes as well as specific health outcomes.[21]

On the third assumption, which is the lynchpin assumption to interventions that involve clinical practice changes, survey research shows that the pediatric practitioner is often the only professional who sees children and their families and is also in a position to assess health and development. As Figure E-1 shows, nearly 90 percent of all young children are seen by a primary care practitioner annually, but fewer than one-third are in any form of formal child care or preschool arrangement. Additionally, there is some research that families do listen to what pediatric practitioners recommend and that anticipatory guidance can affect family practices both on health-

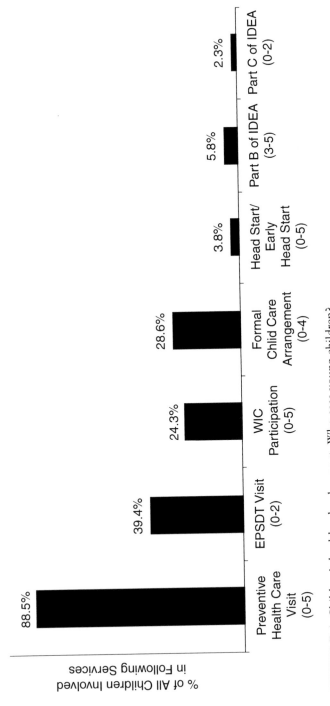

FIGURE E-1 Children's healthy development: Who sees young children?
SOURCE: Hagen et al., 2007.

related and healthy development-related activities. Survey research also provides evidence that current pediatric practice does not take full advantage of these opportunities and that most well-child care falls short of providing recommended screenings, let alone follow-up services, for children, based upon national child health care guidelines.[22]

As the next section of this report shows, there are "exemplary" programs that provide evidence of the potential for such practice changes. Ultimately, as specific initiatives or interventions are developed, the fourth assumption about the value of linking child health care services to other community services needs to be further unpacked, based upon the specific features of that intervention. Ideally an evaluation design would be developed to help answer three questions: (1) Were the planned or desired changes actually feasible and implemented? (2) Did those that were implemented produce both short- and longer-term outcomes for children? and (3) Are the changes replicable, scalable, and subject to diffusion to other child health care practices?[23]

Issues related to disparities that stem from language and cultural incongruities in clinical practice and community resources[24] and to racism (both institutional and individual[25]) must be addressed within the relationships and interactions of the child health care practice and the greater community.

Reducing child health, education, and other disparities by race and ethnicity will require increased efforts to develop such strategies and changed child health practices, coupled with evaluation designs that do not rely upon clinical trials as the sole methodology for attributing causality.

On the fifth assumption relating to the geographic concentration of risk factors, there is strong evidence of the spatial concentration of children of color who experience health disparities (see previous section). There is further evidence of the disproportionate presence of environmental dangers (lead paint, ambient air quality, unsafe housing, and presence of violence) within those neighborhoods. The ability to make significant changes in these environments through policy or initiative, however, remains much more open to question.[26] Some research indicates that parents who are successful in raising their children in these neighborhoods do so by quarantining them from the social and economic connections found within the neighborhood itself and finding support systems elsewhere, rather than building from within.[27] While this may be rational and produce positive results at an individual level, it does not contribute to resolving the underlying community-based problems that must be addressed to produce overall community-wide improvements in child health and development.[28] While these are much larger issues than those related to linking clinical practice strategies to community-building ones, the context for making change within such neighborhoods needs to be recognized as potentially qualitatively as well as quantitatively different than within more advantaged and affluent ones.[29]

Also related to the fifth assumption is strong evidence that social environment matters in healthy child development. This is reflected in parallel research on social capital,[30] resiliency,[31] risk and protective factors,[32] and assets[33]—all of which show that healthy development has social as well as individual determinants. Unless some effective strategies are developed to affect the social environment as well as focus upon individual-level interventions, it is unlikely that disparities in child health and healthy child development outcomes can be appreciably reduced.

On the sixth assumption, that significant improvements in child health and development respond to similar clinical and community-level strategies, the key word is *significantly*. Like most theories of change, this theory and its set of assumptions, as generally stated, clearly has some measure of truth. Given sufficient resources, one would expect some impact on short- or even long-term child health and healthy development outcomes from implementing initiatives based upon this theory. The more important issues are efficiency and extent—how much effect can be produced with what amount of resources, compared with alternative approaches to addressing those disparities.

It is possible to justify even quite substantial investments if they can be shown to reduce disparities through improving outcomes, as the costs of current disparities in both child health and healthy child development outcomes are enormous. Preventable costs related to asthma, obesity, lead poisoning, school dropout, homelessness and lack of employability, and justice system involvement (including costs to society in victimization and incarceration expenses) collectively amount to hundreds of billions, if not trillions of dollars, annually.[34] Developing strategies to reduce health disparities and disparities in healthy child development are warranted from a fiscal as well as a moral perspective. In terms of determining the effects of an initiative relative to the investment of resources made (cost-benefit ratios), the value of looking beyond specific medical health impacts is clear. A child whose asthma has been effectively managed misses fewer days of school and maintains school progress and is likely to have reduced medical costs related to morbidity, fewer compensatory education expenses related to school performance, and improved long-term educational and social outcomes that affect future earnings, tax contributions, and social welfare costs. Taken together, societal savings across these areas may more than justify substantially increased investments in primary and preventive care.[35]

The theory of change presented in this section for the role of child health care practice in contributing to addressing disparities in child health and healthy development helps to establish a framework for designing strategies that link health care to community development, assess their effectiveness and their potential, and learn from them to further improve disparity-reducing policies and practices.

This work does not need to start from scratch, but can build upon experiences and practices in the field. The next section highlights two such approaches.

THE ROLE OF CHILD HEALTH PRACTICE IN REDUCING DISPARITIES IN CHILD HEALTH AND HEALTHY DEVELOPMENT—TWO STRATEGIC APPROACHES

Although research is limited on strategies that incorporate clinical and community-building practices, there is promising evidence that exists around specific programmatic approaches that, explicitly or implicitly, adopt a theory of change similar to that presented in the last section.[36] Two of these—"Help Me Grow" in Connecticut and the "East End Partnership with Families" in Richmond, Virginia—are described here. One takes pediatric well-child practice as its starting point, while the other takes clinical practice within a community health center as its starting point.

Help Me Grow

Help Me Grow is a statewide program in Connecticut to build into young (birth to five) well-child care what pediatrician and program developer Paul Dworkin calls "developmental surveillance." Explicitly based upon the third and fourth assumptions in the theory of change, Help Me Grow itself has three core components.

Training and Support

Help Me Grow incorporates training and support of child health practitioners in broadening their pediatric office visits to incorporate developmental surveillance, starting with asking the question, "Do you have any concerns about how your child is learning, behaving, or developing?" and incorporating appropriate developmental screening tools within the visit. Asked in the practitioner's office, this simple inquiry often elicits a flood of questions from parents about their young child's development and reveals family factors and stressors as well. Help Me Grow has been successful at getting practitioners to ask this question and incorporate developmental surveillance into their routine practices. This has been achieved through short but structured office-based training sessions for practitioners, coupled with a variety of tools for practitioners to use in detecting developmental issues. With this publicly supported training, Help Me Grow also provides practitioners with resources for use in the office, including posters and brochures describing the program and prescription pads for physicians to make referrals to Help Me Grow care coordinators, when warranted. Critically important, Help Me Grow provides an avenue for practitioners to do something when a potential need is identified.

Help Me Grow Care Coordinators

The second core component of Help Me Grow is the care coordinator, who follows up on practitioner referrals or direct family contacts made upon the practitioner's recommendation. Care coordinators talk by phone with parents to further determine child and parental concerns and needs, and then draw upon a continuously developing database of community providers to match parents with services they may need. The federal Individuals with Disabilities Education Act (IDEA) and its early intervention (Part C) program represents one important referral and connection, but many children who may not be eligible for Part C because of age or identified concerns still benefit from developmental health services. On average, care coordinators make seven to eight calls following contact with the practitioner and the family in finding a service match and scheduling a visit or meeting (the amount of time in locating appropriate services is one reason that pediatric practitioners themselves do not generally do this follow-up work outside their established connections with specialists within the medical community). While referrals may be made for additional professional services, many concerns relate to parenting education and support services, including peer support and help. Help Me Grow has found that, in most instances, there are services that parents can access that can provide real help, but finding them for an individual family takes initiative and time. The care coordinators also play the important role of providing information back to the pediatric practitioner on the services that have been matched (so practitioners can follow-up on the next pediatric visit), and conducting follow-up calls with families and programs to ensure they have actually made connections. The care coordinator's work extends beyond simply finding a referral source to scheduling a visit and following up on that visit.

Child Development Community Liaisons

The third core component of Help Me Grow is the child development community liaison, who works closely with the care coordinators in identifying and matching community services. Liaisons work to continuously build the comprehensive community resources database that care coordinators use in their work; they also serve as consultants to the care coordinators on specific cases, in researching for resources that can address specific needs. In addition, the liaisons are on-the-ground networkers across the service-providing community, hosting regular break-fasts or other meetings for community providers to receive guidance and information on selected developmental issues, broaden the overall referral system, and strengthen the networking and relationships across the service community.

Schematically, the Help Me Grow model is shown in Figure 3-5. Help Me Grow also has an evaluation and continuous learning component, one that is considered fundamental to its success.

Initial findings from Help Me Grow have been the subject of a special supplement of the *Journal of Developmental & Behavioral Pediatrics*, and these results tend to confirm the validity of assumptions three and four.[37] Help Me Grow has increased both the identification of young children with developmental problems and their connections to community resources and supports. It has increased child health care providers' understanding and use of other professional services such as Part C and diagnoses and follow-up clinical services for specific mental and developmental health conditions, with at least one follow-up visit achieved for more than 90 percent of all children, according to the most recent report.[38] In addition, it has created a bridge for addressing a variety of more general parental issues and concerns that can affect children's healthy development. Approximately one-quarter of the referrals to care coordinators relate to issues of parenting stress, isolation, or lack of parenting knowledge, or to issues of child discipline and behavior. Approximately the same percentage of follow-up services young children and their families secure through Help Me Grow involve parenting education, parent support groups, and other community programs for parents and their children. Many of the connections Help Me Grow makes are with programs that do not charge fees and involve nonprofessional resources that represent social institutional contacts, reinforcing healthy lifestyles and fostering both child and parental resiliency. Help Me Grow also makes cultural and language connections when locating community resources that families and their young children will feel comfortable with and validated by. It is publicly funded through the state of Connecticut.

East End Partnerships with Families

The East End Partnership with Families in Richmond, Virginia, is another approach to improving children's healthy development, with the Vernon J. Harris Community Center serving as an anchor partner. The Vernon J. Harris Community Center serves as a safety net provider in offering high-quality medical services to children and families who otherwise could not afford such care. At the same time, the center takes a "whole child and whole family" approach to supporting health, recognizing that ensuring good health involves meeting a range of family needs—including

such varied needs as securing housing or rent assistance, supporting rela-
tives providing child care, and providing summer day camp opportunities
for youth.

The East End Partnership includes 10 community partner organizations
that have come to see their role as creating resources and opportunities
that children and their families need for their health and development. The
Parent Resource Network is a critical partner, a parent-led organization
committed to ensuring that family voices in design and family involvement
in implementation is a core aspect of program development.

Central to the East End Partnership with Families is a comprehensive
assessment and client-tracking system that involves common intake and
referral at the Vernon J. Harris Community Center, coupled with care
coordination for the most vulnerable families that helps them to navigate
the array of community agencies they deal with that are designed to provide
them with needed services.

The comprehensive assessment not only identifies needs but also helps
ensure that families know about and can become involved in a wide range
of services, including

- medical care, dental services, and community outreach and assessment services through the Vernon J. Harris Health Center;
- a parent resource network, including advocacy training and support, peer networking, and a variety of support groups, including
  a kinship care support group, a single parents support group, and
  a teen "girl talk" group;
- child guidance services, involving community-based mental health,
  school-based mental health, and preventive mental health services;
  and
- a variety of community programs developed through the partnership's work and partner leadership, based upon needs identified by
  parents and youth and specific opportunities for securing needed
  resources identified by the partnership and its members, including
  such activities as youth drug abuse counseling, teen grief counseling, "raising a reader" programming, obesity prevention programming, and male mentoring and fatherhood programming.

The starting point for the connection with families is the Vernon J.
Harris Health Center and its reputation and standing in the community as
a high-quality and culturally responsive center for providing needed health
services. There are many community health centers with such reputations
in their communities, and many have also developed additional services
and community connections similar to those created in Richmond through
the East End Partnership with Families. They have done so because their

close connections to the children and families they serve have brought such needs and opportunities to their attention, and they have supported resident leaders to advocate for needed services.

The Vernon J. Harris Health Center and the East End Partnership with Families is highlighted as an exemplary but by no means unique effort among community health centers. It is mature and sophisticated, continuously looking for ways to expand the services available to members of its community, often through forging ties and partnerships within a predominantly minority community within a larger political jurisdiction.

As a case in point, the East End Partnership with Families provides substantial evidence for the validity of the fifth assumption—the importance of working within distressed communities—as it has been successful in building social capital, fostering resiliency, and creating a more favorable overall environment for healthy child development within the community.

The growth of the East End Partnership with Families has not been by detailed blueprint; its evolution has been both organic and entrepreneurial. The partnership's successes can be seen in its ability to identify needs and secure resources, but that success truly rests on the infrastructure, support, and leadership it provides. Creating a critical mass of programs, activities, and opportunities that are sufficiently diverse to attract and engage different constituencies may be more important than the provision of specific, discrete professional services (however much they can be tied to clinical need) to improving healthy child development in these neighborhoods.[39]

This ability to activate and motivate its community relates to assumptions, or testable propositions, under the theory of change. While the Vernon J. Harris Community Center and East End Partnership with Families exist in various degrees throughout the country, using this as a model for reducing disparities assumes that there are intentional activities and efforts that can replicate the evolution of the East End Partnership with Families and its level of activity and community engagement. At a minimum, this may involve investing in champions rather than programs. It also assumes that a critical mass of activity will, in fact, change community social capital and community resiliency to produce community improvements related to healthy child development that are more than the sum of individual program parts. At a minimum, testing this assumption requires research methodologies that extend beyond randomized controlled trials, particularly as assignment to a treatment or control group would violate the fundamental, inclusive approach being taken to producing changes in healthy child development.

CONCLUSION, NEXT STEPS, AND
APPROPRIATE METHODOLOGIES

This paper has sought to make the case for changed pediatric clinical practices—particularly around well-child care—to help address disparities in child health and healthy child development by race and ethnicity. The profound disparities in both child health and healthy child development by race and ethnicity cannot be expected to simply disappear without concerted and intentional efforts to address them. They have proved to be persistent in American society and require significant changes in order to address them effectively.

This paper also has asserted that the clinical health community can play an essential, but by no means total or independent, role in reducing these disparities. This clinical role requires both changing clinical health practices (to be more holistic and developmental) and changing ways that clinical practices connect to community (particularly to make effective referrals of patients to community resources and supports).

As case illustrations, the Help Me Grow and East End Partnership with Families examples provide illustrations of organic and holistic approaches to improving healthy child development that start with clinical practice but extend into their communities to produce improvements in healthy child development.

Clearly, there is not a current research base that provides definitive results for efforts that combine individually focused health strategies with community-building efforts that strengthen healthy outcomes on a population level. There is not an established set of protocols and procedures to achieve such ends that can guide practitioners. There is not a research base that has begun to establish the relative size of the effects in reducing disparities that such combined or coordinated efforts might be expected to produce. Compared with the amount of funding expended on research on clinical procedures and drug therapies, the research funding for evaluating such approaches has been miniscule at best. Yet, achieving good outcomes for children requires that current clinical care be improved, and that part of that improvement involves assuring that children and families have ready accesses to a variety of community support services.

More emphasis needs to be provided for this work, which also involves developing evaluation approaches that are rigorous, but that involve different methodologies than randomized controlled trials for attributing causality for at least some aspects of the work.[40] It requires investing in champions who are developing such approaches, involving different approaches when awarding research grants,[41] and giving credence to such efforts and their practitioners within the clinical community. In the end, particularly in the diffusion of such practices, it involves fiscal and regulatory incentives that support them, moving toward broader rather than narrower definitions of what constitutes child health services.[42]

ENDNOTES

1   Halfon, N., and M. Hochstein. 2002. Life course health development: An integrated framework for developing health, policy, and research. *Milbank Quarterly* 80(3):433-479. Forrest, C., and A. Riley. 2004. Childhood origins of adult health: A basis for life-course health policy. *Health Affairs* 23(5):155-164.

2   Family income and socioeconomic status also has strong correlations with a broad variety of child outcomes and with race and ethnicity. *See* Haveman, R., and B. Wolfe. 1994. *Succeeding generations: On the effects of investments in children.* New York: Russell Sage Foundation. There likely is no single etiology to explain all disparities, and there are substantial variations in different child outcomes by different races and ethnicities, independent from income and socioeconomic status, that also need to be addressed.

3   This refers to toxic elements in a broad sense, including environmental exposure to toxic elements (lead paint, chemicals, poor air quality, etc.), exposure to unsafe situations (violence and crime, poor housing, etc.), and presence of a socially toxic environment (social disorganization, absence of positive peer and adult activities, etc.). Garbarino, J. 1995. *Raising children in a socially toxic environment.* San Francisco, CA: Jossey-Bass.

4   In dominant culture, this positive identity often is based on a realistic belief that opportunity exists through personal achievement. The disconnect that minorities may face between that dominant culture belief and their own opportunity (because of institutional racism and/or cultural clashes in undergirding values and expectations) can be cause for alienation, anger, and anomie, all to the detriment of health and healthy development.

5   Views in other parts of the world tend to be more holistic and ecological, particularly within developing countries. The World Health Organization places a very pronounced role on community building as a tool for improving health. The United States itself has a very individualistic political culture, with strong underlying assumptions regarding both personal responsibility and availability of opportunity that tend to view adult outcomes as the result of adult decisions and not external factors. This has led to both health and social interventions and policies that focus upon individual change as opposed to community condition change.

6   The term *child health practitioners* refers to pediatricians, family practitioners, and pediatric nurse practitioners who provide primary care for children.

7   Schor, E. 2007. The future pediatrician: Promoting children's health and development. *Journal of Pediatrics* Nov:S11-S16.

8   This paper will largely use the term *vulnerable neighborhoods* to describe those places where challenges to successfully raising children are greatest. These neighborhoods also have been referred to as "distressed," "disinvested," "poor, tough," or "poor, immigrant, and minority" neighborhoods in the field. This paper also will use the term *children of color* to refer to all children who are not identified as white, non-Hispanic, although Hispanic is considered in the census as a descriptor of origin or ethnicity and not race—and many Hispanics select their race as "white."

9   Horowitz, C., and E. Lawlor. 2007. *Community approaches to addressing health disparities.* Paper for the Institute of Medicine's Roundtable on Racial and Ethnic Health Disparities. *See also* Best, A., D. Stokols, L. Green, S. Leischow, B. Holmes, and K. Buchholz. 2003. An integrative framework for community partnering to translate theory into effective health promotion strategy. *American Journal of Health Promotion* 18(2):168-176.

10 Although entry into early prenatal care is substantially lower in pregnancies among Hispanic women, both low birth weight rates and infant mortality rates are also lower, compared even with pregnancies among white, non-Hispanic women. These data are even more pronounced when controlled for income. A landmark meta-analysis of more than 10,000 international research studies on effective practices in childbirth concluded that "social, psychological, and fiscal supports" were more important to healthy birth outcomes for women without specific medical complications than were clinical visits during pregnancy (and that doulas and nurse midwives produced better birth outcomes than obstetricians for these pregnancies, because they spent more time and provided more social support). Enkin, M., J. Keirse, and I. Chalmers. 1989. *A guide to effective care in pregnancy and childbirth.* Oxford, UK: Oxford University Press. While pregnancy is not necessarily regarded as a medical condition requiring clinical care within Hispanic communities, it is more likely to be treated as a joyous event that involves intensification of attention and support for the woman experiencing pregnancy, such as social and psychological (and to some extent financial) supports. Research also suggests that these more positive birth outcomes among Hispanic women are generally for first-generation immigrants and may not extend to second- and third-generation women whose families and support systems have been acculturated to other practices and roles regarding pregnancy and work.

11 Orzechowski, S., and P. Sepielli. 2003. Net worth and asset ownership of households: 1998 and 2000. *Current Population Reports.* Washington, DC: U.S. Census. Pp. 70-88.

12 Brooks-Gunn, J., G. Duncan, and L. Aber (eds). 1997. *Neighborhood poverty: Volume I.* New York: Russell Sage Foundation. Xue, Y., T. Leventhal, J. Brooks-Gunn, and F. Earls. 2005. Neighborhood residence and mental health problems of 5- to 11-year-olds. *Archives of General Psychiatry* 62(5):554-563.

13 Bruner, C., M. Wright, and S. Tirmizi. (2007). *Village building and school readiness: Closing opportunity gaps in a diverse society.* Des Moines, IA: State Early Childhood Policy Technical Assistance Network. Pp. 5-14.

14 Geomapping of vital records statistics and birth outcomes is increasingly common and shows the spatial concentration of infant mortality, low birth weight, and entry into prenatal care. Elevated blood lead levels also have been geomapped and have extremely high correlations to low-income housing areas of pre-1950s housing. Childhood obesity has even been linked to neighborhoods with high poverty concentrations, lack of access to grocery stores, and absence of safe recreational spaces. The Annie E. Casey Foundation's Making Connections Initiative, working in 10 inner-city neighborhoods across the country, has conducted extensive surveys of residents asking selected questions regarding child health, one of which is identical to the questions from the national health survey regarding childhood asthma. In all Making Connections surveys analyzed (for Denver, Des Moines, Indianapolis, and Oakland), parent-reported asthma prevalence rates among young children were double those of the state as a whole. Bruner, C., and S. Tirmizi. 2007. *Making connections wave II survey and key findings on children healthy and prepared for success in school.* Des Moines, IA: Child and Family Policy Center.

15 Bruner, C., and S. Tirmizi. 2007. *Making connections wave II survey and key findings on children healthy and prepared for success in school.* Des Moines, IA: Child and Family Policy Center.

16 National Scientific Council on the Developing Child. 2005. *Excessive stress disrupts the architecture of the developing brain.* Cambridge, MA: Center on the Developing Child at Harvard University.

17 The Aspen Institute has been a leader in promoting a "theory of change" approach to evaluating comprehensive, community-building initiatives and has produced three useful volumes on this subject. *See* Weiss, C. 1995. Nothing as practical as good theory: Exploring theory-based evaluation for comprehensive community initiatives. In *New approaches to evaluating community initiatives: Concepts, methods, and contexts*, edited by J. Connell, A. Kubisch, L. Schorr, and C. Weiss. New York: Aspen Institute.

18 Genetic factors and individual constitution also contribute to children's health and healthy development but also represent givens, generally not subject to change except through one of the other items on the list.

19 See endnotes 30–33.

20 One such suggested breakdown of the relative contribution to health is constitution (10%), medical care (20%), environmental conditions (20%), and personal factors (50%).

21 Currie, J. 2005. Health disparities and gaps in school readiness. *Future of Children* 15:1.

22 Hagan, J., J. Shaw, and P. Duncan. 2007. *Bright futures: Guidelines for health supervision of infants, children, and adolescents*. Elk Grove Village, IL: American Academy of Pediatrics.

23 Answering these questions requires evaluation methodologies that are both rigorous and appropriate. A promising framework for evaluating comprehensive, systems change initiatives that takes into account their complexity and need for multiple evaluation methodologies while involving rigor in seeking to attribute causality is found in Coffman, J. 2007. *A framework for evaluating systems initiatives.* www.buildinitiative.org (accessed June 9, 2009).

24 For a particularly poignant example, see Fadiman, A. (1997). *The spirit catches you and you fall down: A Hmong child, her American doctors, and the collision of two cultures.* New York: Farrar, Straus, and Giroux.

25 Discussing the underlying effects of racism on child health and healthy development is well beyond the scope of this paper, but the topic deserves a similar provocative discussion as that applied to achievement disparities in education set out in Perry, T. 2003. Up from the parched earth: Toward a theory of African American achievement. In *Young, gifted, and black: Promoting high achievement among African-American students*, edited by T. Perry, C. Steele, and A. Hilliard, III. Boston, MA: Beacon Press. Pp. 1-108. There also is some research that stress produced by contact with discrimination has adverse impacts upon healthy births. Collins, J., R. David, A. Handler, S. Wall, and S. Andres. 2004. Very low birth weight in African American infants: The role of maternal exposure to interpersonal racial discrimination. *American Journal of Public Health* 94(12):2132-2138.

26 Lemann, N. 1994. The myth of community development. *New York Times Sunday Magazine.* January 9, Section 6, 27.

27 Jarrett, R. (1999). Successful parenting in high-risk neighborhoods. *The Future of Children* 9(2):45-50.

28 Bruner, C. 2006. Social service systems reform and poor neighborhoods: What we know and what we need to find out. In *Community change: Theories, practice, and evidence*, edited by K. Fulbright-Anderson, and P. Auspos. New York: Aspen Institute Roundtable on Community Change.

29 Bruner, C. 2006. Village building and school readiness. In *Community change: Theories, practice, and evidence*, edited by K. Fulbright-Anderson, and P. Auspos. New York: Aspen Institute Roundtable on Community Change. Pp. 5-14.

30   Putnam, R. 1993. The prosperous community: Social capital and public life. *The American Prospect* 4 (March 21): 35-42. Putnam, R. 1993. *Making democracy work: Civic traditions in modern Italy.* Princeton, NJ: Princeton University Press.

31   Bernard, B. 1991. Fostering resiliency in kids: Protective factors in the family, school, and community. Portland, OR: Far West Laboratories. Henderson, N. B. Benard, and N. Sharp-Light, eds. 1999. *Resiliency in action: Practical ideas for overcoming risks and building strengths in youth, families, and communities.* San Diego, CA: Resiliency in Action Press.

32   Catalano, R., and D. Hawkins. 1996. The social development model: A theory of antisocial behavior. In *Delinquency and crime: Current theories,* edited by J. Hawkins. New York: Cambridge University Press.

33   Benson, P. 2000. *All kids are our kids: What communities must do to raise caring and responsible children and adolescents.* San Francisco, CA: Jossey-Bass.

34   Guyer, B., S. Ma, H. Grason, K. Frick, A. Perry, and J. McIntosh. (2007). *Investments to promote children's health: A systematic literature review and economic analysis of interventions in the preschool period.* Washington, DC: Partnership for America's Economic Success. Bruner, C. 2001. *A stitch in time.* Washington, DC: Finance Project.

35   The widely cited research on the importance of investing in preschool because of its return on investment is based upon such multiple gains that cover far more than educational impacts. In fact, the educational gains alone would not warrant such investments—it is the social gains (reduced criminal activity, adolescent parenting, etc.) that produce the high rates of return on such investments. *See* Bruner, C. 2006. *Many happy returns.* Des Moines, IA: State Early Childhood Policy Technical Assistance Network.

36   These are only two of many possible programs, selected for illustrative purposes. The American Academy of Pediatric's CATCH program has been working since 1989 to promote better linkages between practice and the community. *See* http://www.jhsph. edu/wchpc/projects/catch.html.

37   Dworkin, P. and J. Bogin, eds. 2006. Help me grow roundtable: Promoting development through child health services. *Journal of Developmental and Behavioral Pediatrics* 27:1S.

38   Hughes, M., M. Damboise. 2007. *Help me grow: 2007 annual evaluation report.* Hartford, CT: Center for Social Research, University of Hartford for the Children's Trust Fund.

39   This is one of five plausible "theories of change" for addressing the needs of children in poor neighborhoods presented more fully in Bruner, C. 2006. Social service systems reform and poor neighborhoods: What we know and what we need to find out. In *Community change: Theories, practice, and evidence,* edited by K. Fulbright-Anderson, and P. Auspos. New York: Aspen Institute Roundtable on Community Change.

40   Coffman, J. 2007. *A framework for evaluating systems initiatives.* Build Initiative. Participatory or empowerment evaluation also has a role in this work, but only if it ultimately also meets some test of attributing causality. This includes the ability for disproof, including disproof of the role of participant-led change as sufficient or necessary for improving healthy child development outcomes.

41   Polansky, N. 1995 (unpublished). *Historical perspective in evaluative research.* Polanski relates the story of Fritz Redl, an imaginative and innovative researcher on developing treatments for disturbed youth. Previously funded by the National Institute of Health, he sought to apply for additional funding, but "came up against a newly erected wall. The applicant was now asked not only whom he wanted to treat, but precisely what the treatment would be, and by what design it would be evaluated so that one could tell whether it differed for those not so treated. ... [Redl needed] funding for a free-wheeling project in which he would try to find ways of approaching heretofore unreachable